STAGING THE MUSICAL

STAGING THE MUSICAL

Organizing, Planning, and Rehearsing the Amateur Production

DAVID GROTE

PRENTICE-HALL, INC.
Englewood Cliffs, New Jersey 07632

Library of Congress Cataloging-in-Publication Data

Grote, David.
    Staging the musical.

    Bibliography.
    Includes index.
    1. Musical revue, comedy, etc.—Production and
direction. I. Title.
MT955.G77 1986   782.81′07′1   85-28223
ISBN 0-13-840182-9

Printed in the United States of America.
10 9 8 7 6 5 4 3 2 1

Contents

Contents

Preface

Everything in this book is based on a simple assumption: Every amateur production of a musical can be a good one. Most groups can not only do musicals but can do them well.

In general, people tend to think that amateur productions of musicals must be mediocre at best. This need not be true. If productions are not as good as they should be, it is rarely due to lack of performing talent. In most places, talent is there. What's missing is everything else—experience, skill, and most of all preparation, planning, and organization. Talent alone cannot make a good musical production; neither can talent combined only with money. But talent, combined with careful organization and preparation, can. The disorganization, the bitter infighting, the disappointment, and the ulcers that usually accompany such productions are not essential parts of the process.

It would be wonderful if life were like a Mickey Rooney movie, if lots of energy were all we needed for a great musical show. Unfortunately, staging a musical well is the most complex process in the theater. It requires months of preparation, complex organizational procedures, legal, financial, and personal commitments, detailed preparation and rehearsal, and much experience and skill on the part of an enormous number of different persons. Problems in such a complex process can never be eliminated. *But they can be kept to a minimum.* This book is intended to help people with talent make efficient use of that talent by indicating typical problem areas and suggesting ways to avoid or minimize those problems.

Although the book is about "putting on a show," it deals primarily with those things that must normally be learned the hard way, if at all. It won't explain how to act or how to sing and dance; it assumes that most of the people who are likely to read this will already know how to do at least one of those things with some degree of competence. It will explain how to get organized, how to understand the weird traditions and conventions of the American musical comedy, how to use those traditions in planning and preparing, and how to keep a production functioning in rehearsal so that all the available talent can be seen to best advantage.

The musical is not only the most complex but also the most popular form of American theatre. It demands great skill, but it can and should give great pleasure both to the audience *and* to the performers. It is possible to do musicals, do them well, use local talent, make the most of limited budgets, and still stay sane, make a profit (however small), and keep all the people involved speaking to one another after the show is finished. This book describes one practical way to do that.

This book could not have been completed without the kind cooperation of the following people to whom I am most grateful: Robert Titlow, Jim Jester, John Faust, Ronn Goswick, Barbara Lynch, Cathy Henry, Deborah Slate, Allen B. Whitehead, Jack Shannon, Dean Hess, Scott Quintard, Tom Orr, James Culley, and Susan Archibald Grote. In addition, I want to thank the hundreds of people, far too numerous to name, with whom I have worked over the years, who provided both the problems and the solutions that taught me what I have learned about musicals, and most especially Louise Thomas, without whose bravery I should never have begun, and Mike Mc-Querrey, whose talent and musicianship demonstrated how collaboration should and could work.

STAGING THE MUSICAL

1

Overture

There's nothing like a musical. Nothing in the theatre quite matches that thrill of anticipation and exhilaration when the house lights dim and the overture begins. It's a magical moment, a promise that something wonderful is about to happen. And there's nothing quite like the aura of happiness and good feeling that an audience projects when that promise is fulfilled by a good musical in a good production, whether professional or amateur.

Thus, it should come as no surprise that both individuals and organizations in every age group and in every community across the country, no matter how small, want to see or to produce their own musicals. Each year, it seems, the number of amateur musical productions increases. High schools, community theatres, and independent groups are all attracted to the special excitement of the American musical.

Unfortunately, it's a long way from the moment someone is inspired to stage a musical to the moment the audience hears the overture on opening night, and the process of planning properly and rehearsing well is long and complex. A good musical production demands all the skills, energy, and commitment of any theatrical production, plus an enormous number of additional requirements that are unique to the musical itself.

In the chapters that follow, we will examine those unique requirements in order to suggest ways to surmount the challenges, even if this is your first musical production, and obtain the rewards that accompany a truly satisfying quality performance.

WHY DO A MUSICAL?

The attractions of musical productions are so great and so generally understood that we need mention them only briefly.

Almost all performing groups like musicals for the following reasons:

- They are well known.
- They draw large audiences in relation to other kinds of theatrical productions.
- They raise more money than other kinds of theatrical productions.
- They offer roles for large numbers of performers.
- They offer roles for performers with a variety of skills and experiences.
- They involve large portions of the community.
- They carry a lot of status and draw much favorable local attention and publicity.

School teachers and administrators seem particularly attracted to musicals for additional reasons. Because the casts are large and the production skills so varied, the musical can use many different types of students whose talents could not otherwise ever be combined into a single project. In turn, all that student involvement usually leads to both enormous audiences and much parental support, which has made the school musical one of the major public relations tools of the modern high school principal (second only to sports in most school situations). As a result, teachers are not only allowed but often assigned to produce them. The practice is so successful that it is now spreading down into the junior high- and elementary-school level.

In addition, performers like musicals for any number of individualized reasons, not the least of which is the demand for several different skills. No matter how much we admire our actors, the fact remains that for most Americans, performing "talent" means singing or dancing, or both. Thus, until we have done a musical, there is the feeling that we haven't really tested or demonstrated our talent. In a musical, performers also get to deal with some of the most interesting popular music in our culture and usually get lots of applause and public recognition. Even people who don't want to solo are attracted because musicals offer so many roles of so many different sizes; people who want to be on stage but who would never work up their nerve for a large role can get experience and security in the chorus or in one of the smaller roles.

All these different attractions mean that we need not devote a great deal of space to convincing you that a musical production might be a good thing for you or your group. The question is, What is the best way to go about producing the musical so that you and your organization will realize all the potential advantages of that production?

CAN YOU DO A MUSICAL?

Unfortunately, the musical does not always turn out as dreamed. Staging a musical production is an enormous amount of work requiring a number of different skills, and there are hundreds of different ways in which the process can go wrong.

In the following chapters, we will examine most of the potential problems and solutions, beginning with the selection of a show that is suited to your own particular needs, facilities, and skills. Then we will follow a typical production process for that show, examining ways to understand the unique conventions and performing demands of musicals in general and your show in particular, how to establish a sound budget for the production, and how to organize and coordinate the enormous staff needed for your show so that rehearsals can begin. Then we will look at the procedures and problems of casting, rehearsing, and solving the unique technical staging problems of most musicals.

Many people who want to do musicals jump in without ever considering these problems, and as a result wear themselves out trying to do too many things at once or things that don't work. Many others look at all these potential problems and wonder if it's really worth it or if they can ever find people with the many different skills needed. Still others want to do musicals, but they have been "burned" by bad experiences in other productions and have begun to think that such pain and anguish is an essential part of the process. Still others want to do musicals, but only if they can be sure of doing them better than anyone has ever done them in their community.

The ideas, procedures, and suggestions that follow are addressed in some way to all these people. Once your production is under way, no one person can or should do all of the work described here, but everyone who begins the production process should understand the full process in order to use the skills and talents of all available persons as productively as possible.

If you have never staged a musical before—let's say you are a speech or drama teacher or a choral director whose principal has just suggested rather strongly that a musical would be a nice thing for you to direct this spring—this book will tell you how to pick a show, how to get organized, what help to look for from other people, and what problems to anticipate.

If you are one of those "other people" called on to help in a production, it will help you organize a specific job within the production.

If you have worked in some capacity on other musicals, this will help you take on a new job or suggest how some of the problems you faced in the past can be avoided in future productions.

If you are a member of the production staff, this will help you understand the needs and the terminology used by others on the staff, so that you can communicate and coordinate with each other toward a single goal—the finished production.

If you are a board member of a community theatre or a principal of a school, this will introduce you to the complexity of the process that is often hidden from the view of the people who supervise the production, so that you can better understand what is happening and what you are expecting others to accomplish.

If you are a performer, this will help you understand why things are done the way they are often done.

Most important, what follows should help simplify the day-to-day life of musical production and make it more productive. We want to do musicals because they are good for us, for our organizations, and for our communities. The only way this really happens, however, is if the productions themselves are good ones. Everyone *can* do good productions, but no one does them by accident; good musical productions are definitely made, not born. It's a long, difficult process but an unusually exciting and rewarding one as well, often the most exciting and rewarding in all modern theatre.

A VAMP FOR DEFINITION

Everyone knows what a musical is, and yet it is almost impossible to come up with a clear definition. There are a lot of different kinds of shows that people call musicals, and specialists may call these anything from *opera* to *melodrama*, with *opera seria, comic opera, ballad opera, folk opera, operetta, zarzuela, light opera, musical comedy, musical revue, musical extravaganza, musical theatre, play with music, music drama, the English pantomime, the vaudeville, the burlesque* (as distinct from *Vaudeville* and *Burlesque*), and most recently something called *performance art* all somewhere in between. All these musicals use song in some kind of theatrical or dramatic context, but no two sets of definitions agree: Is *The Pirates of Penzance* an operetta, a comic opera, a burlesque, or a musical comedy? Is *Porgy and Bess* a musical, an operetta, a folk opera, or an opera?

For our purposes, we will leave specific definitions to the specialist and will consider a musical to be essentially any show that a typical nonspecialist would call a musical. For the most part, this means shows that include the following: (1) both music and dialogue, (2) performers who portray some particular kind of character rather than appearing as themselves, and (3) music and dance in the popular idiom. The term also implies shows written around 1940 or thereafter. During this period, people called these shows *musical comedies*, even though a number of them are quite serious in tone, so we will use the slightly less misleading general term *musical*.

The operetta as it is generally understood falls for the most part within this definition. With a few exceptions, noted in Chapter 3 and in the discussion on page 196, it shares the same performance conventions (one major study of the operetta defines it simply as a musical comedy written before 1930). In recent years most operettas have fallen into obscurity, primarily because the styles of popular music have changed so enormously, but the planning, rehearsing, and production techniques that we will discuss can be readily applied to them as well.

Thus, when we use the term, although most of the specific examples will come from what many now consider a "golden age"—beginning with *Oklahoma!* and continuing through *Fiddler on the Roof*—some examples will come from shows as early as the works of Gilbert and Sullivan and as recent as *Sunday in the Park with George*. (A more detailed illustration of the variety of shows included in the term can be seen in the discussion beginning on page 192.

Having thus narrowed our topic to some degree, let's return to the process of staging the musicals themselves, beginning with the selection of a show for production.

2

Show Selection

In the course of production for your musical you will make many important decisions, but none will be more important than the first one— selecting the show itself. Budgeting, casting, rehearsal planning and operation, and in many cases even staffing decisions will be determined or limited by this crucial decision.

HOW NOT TO DO IT

Many school and community groups encounter production problems because they fail to take enough care in their initial selection. In general, there are three misguided approaches, all with significant drawbacks.

The "What's Famous?" Approach

For many groups, the term *musical* means one of two things: recent Broadway shows or movies, or the all-time standards that "everybody" does on a regular basis. So when someone says, "Let's do a musical," the group selects a famous name, announces auditions, and orders scripts. Then the chaos begins, because they had no idea what they were letting themselves in for.

The "I Just Saw a Great Show!" Approach

In this approach, one or two people describe a terrific show they just saw (or heard on a cast album) until everyone else wants to do the show, too.

In almost all cases, this leads to problems for a very simple reason: The most exciting or impressive part of a professional production is most often the one part of the production that is most difficult for amateur groups to reproduce. *Forty-Second Street* has some fascinating tap-dance numbers, but how many organizations can get two dozen professional-level tap dancers, much less afford the sets that surround them? People who see *Evita* and come back home eager to produce it are generally most excited by the mobile movie-screen effects, the one part of the show almost no amateur group could afford to do. This does not mean that you should not consider the original productions of shows, but it does mean that you should try to separate the show itself from the production you have seen elsewhere. Don't get so carried away that you forget the impossibility of doing it the same way even in the best of circumstances.

The "What Does So-and-So Want to Play?" Approach

In this approach, a show is selected simply because one or two people want to play particular roles, and they exert so much pressure that the group eventually agrees to the production.

This leads to an incredible number of problems. First, a *star vehicle* by definition is a show in which almost all the "good stuff" is given to one or two people, which makes it hard to find people to play all those thankless smaller roles. Second, when people are fascinated by individual roles, they tend not to consider the production difficulties of the show as a whole. People who think of playing only Mama Rose in *Gypsy*, for example, fail to consider how many sets, special effects, and costs are involved in the rest of the show. Third, this approach increases the possibility of personal conflicts during the rehearsal period. If Ms. X spent a year lobbying for *My Fair Lady*, she will expect not only to play Eliza but also to see that she is not overshadowed by anyone else on stage while she is performing. Before rehearsals are finished, she will have made life miserable for anyone who disagreed with her about anything that affected her vision of the show. This kind of thinking, which leads to unnecessary conflicts within the cast and with the production staff, is an inadequate and potentially dangerous reason for selecting a script.

There are, however, some valid factors in these three approaches—the show you pick must have some attraction for the cast and the audience. But these approaches cover only a few of the considerations you must deal with when selecting a show for production. At a practical level, they are not even the most important considerations. No matter how much you may love a particular show, no matter how popular the show might be, if your organization cannot mount the production well at this time, you should not do it. After all, how can you let yourself do something you love in any but the best possible way?

This does not mean that you should never do the show, nor does it even imply that amateurs should not do "professional" musicals. It merely means that some shows are more suited to your group, facility, budget, and skills than are others. Because you are doing the show, at least in part, for the pleasure and excitement of doing it well, then you should seek to find the best available script for your circumstances. As future circumstances change, the kinds of scripts you select will change. Sooner or later, if you keep doing shows, you will get the chance to work on your favorite musical. Until then, however, we must focus on a way to select the best available show for a particular situation at a particular time. Such a selection demands a great deal of time, effort, and study.

WHO DECIDES?

One of the most complex parts of this time, effort, and study comes at the very beginning, when the decision-making starts. Someone has to select the script for production. In most organizations, this decision is in effect made by one or two people—the most powerful teacher at the school, the most influential members of the community theatre board of directors, and the like—but such a procedure does not always work to advantage.

Ideally, the people who are responsible for staging the show should select the show. Who better understands the potential strengths and weaknesses of scripts under consideration than the various directors and designers who will ultimately stage the show? At the same time, there must be opportunity for some input and even the possibility of veto by the administrative staff when the selection seems to disagree with the nature, image, or capabilities of the organization as a whole. In general, however, more groups err in play selection by ignoring the expertise of experienced creative people than by taking on an ambitious work because the various directors enthusiastically recommended it.

In practice, play selection demands that most dreaded of all theatrical institutions, the committee. At the school level, this committee should be quite small, consisting of the two or three teachers who will eventually stage the show. At the community theatre level, however, there is usually a committee formed for the express purpose of choosing a show or several shows for a season.

A good selection committee should have people who represent several different viewpoints. Its members should include at least one person with each of the following areas of expertise:

- Reading and staging scripts
- Reading and teaching or leading music
- Dancing and/or dealing with local dance talent
- Building, budgeting, and/or renting scenery and costumes
- Organizational facilities and community relations

As we shall see in the following process, each of these points of expertise will be essential at some point in the decision-making process.

It is important that this committee be kept to a practical size. Any group larger than five will probably be too awkward to make decisions within the time usually available.

Schools often face a particular problem in play selection: the interference of the principal, headmaster, or president of the school. This is a sensitive area. In a school, the chief administrator does have a veto power over all play selection, whether such power is useful or not, and there is no point in wishing it were not so. This power has been established by long tradition and upheld by state and federal courts in the past decade. How this power is exercised will vary from school to school, depending on the relations between the staff and the administrator involved. The key point for a selection committee to establish, however, is that such authority must be limited to a veto power. Do not let the administrator pick the musical and then assign staff to stage it. This is always disastrous. Administrators can and will often veto a selection for various reasons usually related to public relations rather than artistic considerations. But they need not exercise any additional participation in the selection process.

MAKING THE SELECTION

In almost all instances, you must rent or purchase copies of the scripts and pay production royalties to an agency that represents and publishes the musicals. Except in those few cases such as a new script (when you may need to deal directly with the writers or their agent), the overwhelming majority of shows will be contracted from a handful of companies that specialize in such materials. These agencies are described beginning on page 183.

Write to each of the agencies offering the kind of material in which your group is interested and ask for information or catalogs. They will quickly place you on their regular mailing lists and send you regular updates and revisions; in some cases, it will seem as if you receive something from them every week. Once those catalogs have arrived, convene the committee and begin the process of selection.

Step 1:
Obtain Copies for Examination

Examine the various catalogs and look for shows described that might be of interest to your group. Remember that catalog descriptions are advertisements and are designed with sales as their goal. Don't let a good description or a famous name lure you into a purchase without first carefully examining the product—the complete script and score of the show.

Agencies that rent rather than sell scripts or music parts will send you *perusal copies* for examination, usually for two weeks, for the cost of the postage involved and, sometimes, a small deposit. Agencies that do not rent materials will require that you buy examination copies, but the cost is not particularly outrageous and generally little more than the postage and insurance for rental materials.

Recordings of many shows are also available, but even if you have a cast album, always request a perusal copy of the score. In almost all cases there are significant differences between the recordings and the music used in the show. Many numbers are often modified or omitted entirely in the recordings, and dance music is almost always shortened.

Examine several different scripts at the same time, but don't try to read every musical you can think of. Remember that eventually everyone on the committee must examine the script for each work under consideration, and do not order more copies than the group could consider in the typical two-week examination period. (If you are purchasing copies, of course you will have longer to consider them and may read more widely.) If the first shows you examine are not suitable, you may always order and examine others. The only limits are the amount of time available for the selection process and your budget for postage or examination copies.

If you are pressed for time, you may also request royalty information when you request perusal copies (see Step 6 below).

Step 2:
Examine the Scripts Carefully

As soon as perusal copies arrive, circulate them among all the members of the committee. *Read them.* Many groups tend to skimp on this process. The music director looks at the score only, leaving the "story" to the stage director, and the dance director settles for a quick summary of the kinds of dances needed, ignoring the rest of the script. Other committees split the scripts up, with each person making a report on one script. Such methods defeat the purpose of the selection committee. Unless every person involved in the decision reads the script, the different viewpoints and expertise of all the people will be wasted.

In the same way, be sure that the nonmusical people have all heard the music and at least looked at the score. A cast album may be helpful here, but if you intend to perform without a full orchestra, as many groups must do, the album can be positively misleading. A modern, heavily orchestrated show like *A Little Night Music, Promises, Promises*, or *The Wiz* will sound completely different when that orchestration is reduced or eliminated. In such a case, it is better to assemble the group to hear someone play at least parts of the score on piano than to listen to recordings. This will give you an excellent idea of the actual sound you are likely to hear on stage.

Step 3:
Form a Basic Impression of the Scripts

While reading through the scripts and reading or listening to the scores, consider these basic questions.

Do you like the show?

Every dramatic presentation requires a lot of work; any musical requires more. Most of this work will be done by volunteers, who are very much like the people selecting the show. Volunteers work harder, more often, and more creatively when they like the material. The audience must like the show eventually, but the staff and cast must like it from the beginning, or you will have difficulty finding a cast and staff.

This does not necessarily mean the show should be familiar, although people often like what they know has been proven in other places. It does mean the material should be good, in whatever way you choose to define good. People must devote their time, their work, often their money, and their nerves to present the show, and they want to be able to hold their heads up with pride in the community once the show has been seen. All this is easier if they believe in the value, quality, and pleasure of the material itself.

It is extremely important that all the people who select the show ask this question so that a number of different viewpoints are considered. A show that the music director loves and the stage director hates will not be one of the group's best efforts.

Will your audience like the show?

This is an impossible question to answer and a terribly misleading one, yet it must be considered. Musicals cost money and require large resources. If the bodies don't come to the ticket window, dollar bills in hand, everyone is going to have problems.

At the same time, nothing is more depressing to watch than a show thrown up without spirit, imagination, or sincerity, just because the group thought the audience would be stupid enough to like it. This happens most often in schools, where many people choose material on the sole criterion that it is unlikely to upset anyone in the community. However, many a community group has made the same mistake while trying to balance a season, to find a hit to compensate for some low attendance on other shows, or to start out a new group with a guaranteed hit.

Problems with this question arise because almost all of us have learned to think of the audience as a negative force, rather than as the ultimate reason for the existence of the theatrical production. Perhaps because we have lived with television programing for so long, we have come to think of the audience as somehow ignorant, especially in artistic matters. They are not. They are people just like the people who will be working on the show. They have interests and concerns and opinions, just as do the people who will select the show. They may not have the same artistic background as theatre professionals or dedicated amateurs, but that does not affect their ability to respond as an audience. Just as you do not need to be a trained mechanic to enjoy the way a good car feels when you drive it, they need not have music or theatre degrees to enjoy a good theatrical production. The fascinating thing about the theatre is that productions are written to communicate with many different kinds of people of many different backgrounds who share the production together at the same time. Pleasing that audience is not the same thing as looking for the lowest common denominator. It means finding material that can seize their interest, satisfy their curiosity, and engage their spirits in some way, and then doing the material so well that their interest is in fact engaged throughout the performance.

It also helps to remember that most groups know who will come to see the show and that most of those people will come no matter what show you select. Only general community theatre groups tend to draw from the community at large, and then only after they are well established; such groups must depend on a combination of their own reputation and the fame of the title to attract large audiences. But all other groups depend primarily on friends, relatives, and general acquaintances of cast members or people who support the sponsoring organization. The fame of the title may affect their attendance to some minor extent, but for most productions they will show up no matter what is being produced. A show that they will like is simply a show that will interest and entertain them once they take their seats, not a show that they already like because they have seen it somewhere else or wish they had seen it somewhere else. Look for that in your consideration, not for what names might be most attractive in a publicity campaign.

Where will you be performing?

There are a number of important practical points about the performance location that must eventually be considered before the selection is complete (see Step 5), but before you go any further with a particular script, you must consider the ambiance of your eventual performance site.

For example, how large is it? Large auditoriums with lots of seats tend to encourage—even demand—large shows, or shows that feel large. This has little to do with potential audience size. *Godspell*, for example, could fill large theatres in most communities across the country. But the show itself feels small and intimate. Trying to perform it in a 2500-seat auditorium or outdoor theatre would completely destroy the intimate, personal feeling that is so essential to the success of the show. In the same way, *My Fair Lady* is actually a very small show, with most of the stage time devoted to two- and three-person conversation. Yet the show feels big and important and seems to need impressive, large surroundings for successful production.

Another factor is the nature of the community's use of the building. What other organizations use the theatre, and for what purpose? How do people see the building? If this is the place where all the major local events happen, then you want the show to be something just as important. If it is associated with serious artistic endeavor, then you would want to do something that suggests you are involved in such an endeavor.

In many cases, the building itself will preclude the use of some material. If you are renting the hall of the First Baptist Church, you would not want to do *The Best Little Whorehouse in Texas*, even though your organization may have nothing to do with the church itself, nor would you want to do the same show in the local high school auditorium, even if you are a community theatre group merely renting the facility. Each facility carries important associations that all groups using the space must share. These must be considered as you begin to examine the script.

FIRST ELIMINATION

If the majority of the selection committee agrees that any script fails to meet any of the three basic criteria in Step 3, then that script can be eliminated from further consideration. The next step is quite complex and detailed, and there is no reason to take the time to consider all the factors in it if you have a script that no one likes to begin with or that would obviously be unsuitable for your performing space.

Step 4:
Evaluate the Script

From the remaining scripts under consideration, examine the following points. Complete answers to each will require the combined expertise of all the people on the selection committee, so this evaluation is usually best done in discussion.

What are the cast requirements?

Analyzing cast requirements requires more than a quick look at the cast list. Determine for each role the kind of songs to be sung, the amount and kind of dancing, if any, required, the need for any specialized performance skills such as accents, magic tricks, and so forth.

Also determine whether any roles can be doubled, how many people must be in the chorus, and whether the singers and dancers are separate groups or must be able to do both.

What are the staging requirements?

At this point you need not solve all the technical problems of the show; however, you do need to recognize what those problems are. These include such things as the number of different stage settings, costumes, and props required, and the general complexity of each of those items.

Be careful at this time to confine your evaluation to the actual requirements of the show, which are not always the same things as were done in New York or in other productions you have seen. There are often better and cheaper ways to stage most shows than the way they were originally staged in New York.

Be especially alert to little details that might be overlooked. For example, *My Fair Lady* can be done relatively easily with a few drops and nice period costumes, most of which are easily available from rental companies. But the show has four different sets that require *accurate* and *different* period antique furniture indicative of wealth. Two of these sets are complete rooms. Such requirements can cause far more difficulty than all other production requirements combined.

What kind of space will be needed?

Consider the amount of space needed on stage for the largest scenes, for the dancers to dance, for the crowds to maneuver, and so on. Also consider how much space you will need backstage while these large groups maneuver into position before or after their entrances. Then consider the space you will need both for putting the scenery on stage and storing it when it is off.

Step 5:
Evaluate Your Resources

Once you have answered the questions in Step 4, discuss and consider your group's ability to deal with those requirements.

Can you find the talent?

It is not necessary to cast the show before you select it. At the same time, it would be foolish to try to do *A Chorus Line* when there are no dancers available.

This is a genuine problem for schools and other groups that must work from a limited talent pool. In any given school, there will be only a few singers of solo quality for most Broadway-styled scores, and only a handful of dancers (if that many) with serious dance training. Most of those people are known before auditions because they already sing with the choir or dance with the dance classes. Thus, it is possible for the selection committee to estimate whether the organization can in fact find singers or dancers to fit the needs of the show.

In community groups it is much harder to guess what talent might be available. For the most part, the only people the members of the committee will know will be people who have been associated with other shows. This leads to a tendency to pick the same old shows over and over because people know they can be cast. But it's a very rare community that doesn't have an enormous untapped talent pool whose members are capable of playing many roles in many different shows. All they're waiting for is a chance.

Most groups worry about the wrong roles in a show. Although it might sound cynical, most principal roles in musicals are written for either stars or very specific types, often to disguise the limited talents of the original performers; thus, they often require less actual talent than the supporting roles. If you can get people to auditions, you will usually find people to play the principals, no matter what the show.

Casting problems are going to come among the supporting roles. For example, most groups auditioning for *Oklahoma!* will find a dozen Laureys and Curleys. What they usually won't find are the dancers.

Will has to be spectacularly good, all the cowboys have to be reasonably competent, and you need two solo male dancers to double for Curly and Jud in the dream dances. This is why you must consider carefully the script requirements for *all* the roles in the production before making a decision. Don't commit to a show that demands more than your talent pool can provide; there is no point in starting on a show unless you intend to do it well.

Can your facility meet the practical requirements?

Do the stage and auditorium you intend to use have room for all the scenery, props, costumes, and performers that the script requires? Do they have the equipment necessary to handle the electrical and scenic requirements, especially spotlights? Is there available power for additional lighting equipment and some arrangement for hanging and using scenery drops? Remember, you need not solve the problems the same way as done in New York, but you must still be able to solve the problems.

Are the audience areas large enough to hold the audience you will need to pay for the production? This is a circular question, but you must at least consider it. You cannot know how much the show will cost until a complete budget is made (see Chapter 4), and you cannot plan a budget until you have selected the show. In the same way, you cannot know how many people will actually want to see the show until the show is finished. But if you want to do one of the expensive, spectacular musicals, you must have a lot of seating space or run the show for many nights in order to recoup expenses. At the same time, larger houses lead to their own problems: Royalties increase as the seating increases and/or ticket prices rise; larger stages require more massive, spectacular scenery and costumes, which in turn cost more money; the spiral goes on forever. But you must pool all your understanding and make an educated guess at whether there is any hope of actually breaking even on a production that has the basic requirements you have found.

Can the organization
itself handle the show?

Most groups tend to underestimate themselves in this area, but it is important to evaluate seriously the organization's situation before embarking on a particular show. Consider each of the following factors.

Financial stability There are a number of ways to approach this issue, but they all eventually boil down to a single question: What happens if the audience you need doesn't come? Most people start musicals in the assumption that they will make money to be used for supporting charities, covering deficits from more serious shows, or seeding the next production. But the number of well-done musicals I have seen anywhere that have made any significant profit is very small, and almost all those were either *Godspell, Charlie Brown,* or *The Fantasticks*. With planning and care, most groups can break even or make a small profit, but sometimes you may misjudge. Starting a musical is not unlike sitting down at the Friday-night poker game. You must ask how much you can afford to lose. If you cannot risk large sums of money, then don't be tempted by shows that will cost large sums of money to produce.

Resources Many organizations can cut their expenses by having access to a backlog of resources. Some of these come from the community and include various kinds of contributions that may significantly reduce the cost of the show. (These are discussed in Chapter 4.) Others come from the organization itself. Most important of these is a rent-free theatre building. Others include such varied items as old drops from previous productions that can be repainted, extensive costumes in storage that might be suitable for a production, or access to or ownership of a well-equipped scene shop where scenery can be constructed more cheaply than it can be rented. Everything you already have, from sound systems to paint buckets, will be a help in making a script possible and practical. Everything you don't have will be a financial drain on the production.

Organizational stability Can the organization itself cope with the needs of a particular musical? We know that the organization thinks it can cope with *a* musical, or you would not be in the selection stage, but some musicals put more strain than others on the facilities and the personal relationships within the organization. For example, in a school, can the stage be reserved for all the rehearsals needed? In many schools, the stage is in the gym. When the school puts on a play, the actors rehearse in classrooms because the basketball team is in the gym. In a musical, where dancers in particular need the full space of the stage to rehearse, can the stage be given to them, or a space as large with a wooden floor (that is, the gym floor itself) for rehearsals? Where will the basketball or volleyball team go? If you are unable to get that rehearsal space, you may have to eliminate a show that requires any significant number of dance routines.

Much more difficult is the question of organizational skill. Is your organization likely to find the staff people with the necessary skills? If, for example, the play requires an orchestra of good musical quality, are you likely to find skilled orchestra players? If you must hire them, can you afford them? If this is one of the newer shows that demands a number of elelctronic instruments and players, are you likely to find them? If you need a classically oriented dance director, as with *Carousel,* are such people available in the community? Will you have to hire people or even bring in professional people from out of town? Are you committed to working with particular staff members, as in a school that must use specific teachers and students with limited skills in certain areas essential to the show? All such similar factors must be considered.

Some groups underestimate their skill; others overestimate it. It is a hard area in which to give advice. For the most part, any group should be willing to take some chances in any production. Long after people have officially left school, they still need to learn, and theatrical people thrive on good new challenges. But a group with no choreographer should not do *A Chorus Line* or *Dancin'* just because it is an exciting challenge. Somewhere down the road there must be the possibility of a good production.

Community response Finally, you must consider probable community response. Part of this is financial: Will people want to come and buy tickets? But part of it has to deal with community relations in general. Of necessity, school teachers are used to dealing with this question, but all groups must consider it at some time. Do you want your organization associated in the mind of the community at large with this particular show? Many shows can be modified to some extent to meet community standards (see Chapter 5), but other shows by their very nature or reputation will cause problems or misconceptions in the community, no matter how modified.

For example, one of the four or five most brilliant productions of any kind that I have seen was a production of *Hair*. It is my firm belief that if you changed the title to *Fun in the Park*, cut out the use of about a dozen words, and turned out the lights two seconds sooner at the end of the first act, you would have a show that would not upset anyone in almost any community. Yet, you will never get the chance to do that. The title *Hair* is so widely associated with what is regarded as a "dirty" show that most groups would face enormous community outrage just by putting up the posters.

Many other shows have similar problems: *Gypsy* because one of its heroines is a stripper, *Pippin* because of its fame as a sexy show in New York, *Best Little Whorehouse in Texas* for obvious reasons, *Threepenny Opera* because it was written by a well-known avowed Communist. Many groups in many communities must simply eliminate such shows from consideration or risk an enormous amount of negative local publicity.

Even when the community may have no negative preconceptions about the show, the content of the show may be such that you do not wish to be associated with it. I find *Grease* personally distressing, for example, because its moral is that a young girl can't find happiness until she drops out of school and loses her virginity. Although this is expressed with a great deal of vigor and fun, it is not a point that I believe is valid. Thus, I would be unlikely to do the show anywhere and would never do the show in a school. Other people do not share that attitude, as may be seen by the number of school productions of *Grease*, but it is a factor to be considered by any group. You must ask, "What impression will this show give to an attentive audience?" Then ask, "Do we want our group to be associated with such an impression?"

Educational value School groups should consider a unique factor that most other groups need not think about when selecting their shows: What will the students learn while doing the show? Will it teach them anything they need to know? Will it teach them anything they don't already know? In all cases, there will be some theatrical, musical, or performing skills to be learned by some of the students. In some cases, such as *1776*, the subject matter of the musical may be of serious educational value, but in most shows that will not be true. Are there enough parts for a number of different students to work and learn in? Is the show or the music or the technical production different from the kind of things the students have already done in their educational experience? Will we simply get a show on, or will we get a show on and teach and learn something at the same time?

SECOND ELIMINATION

After detailed discussion of these points among all the members of the selection committee, some of the scripts under consideration may be eliminated. In not a few cases, all the scripts you first requested will be eliminated, and you must start again. Eventually, however, you will find that you can narrow down your options to two or three shows, all of which are attractive to most of the committee and within the financial and practical range of the organization at this time.

Now you may move to the final step in the selection process.

Step 6:
Determine the Royalty and Rental Fees

If you have followed the foregoing procedure, you will have narrowed the final selection down to two or three scripts, each of which has different attractions. Before a final decision can be reached, one more factor must be considered.

Royalty   Royalty is a fee paid for the right to present someone else's work. For payment of such a fee, the copyright holder, or his or her agent, grants specifically defined rights to perform the work at a particular time and place. Such fees are split in various ways among the original writers, agents, publishers, producers, and directors of the original production of the show. In general, the royalty fee will be based on some percentage of the gross revenue a production will earn. However, for almost all amateur productions, agents will estimate your income and then quote you a fixed fee because there is no practical way for them to audit your statements of gross income.

Most shows require rental fees, which are paid for the use of rehearsal materials. Rental fees include scripts, musical parts for the singers, scores for accompanists and conductors, and parts for the orchestra. In some cases, fees also include publicity kits, but these can also be rented separately. These fees are usually fixed and will be the same for all groups, no matter what the expected gross income.

However, your rental fees will almost always cost more than first expected. Normally, the rental fee will be quoted for a basic kit, which includes librettos for all the speaking roles and music parts for all the same roles and a fixed number of chorus members. In almost all cases, you will need additional copies of materials, which will require additional fees. If you have a larger chorus, you will need extra music parts. The basic kit will usually include only one or two piano scores, but you will need one for each pianist, one for the conductor, another for the music director, and you should provide one for the stage director and the choreographer to use in their planning as well. If there are extensive cues in musical numbers, the stage manager will also need one. Extra librettos will be needed for each of the directors, and it never hurts to have one or two extra for publicity people and for cast members who will temporarily misplace their own. Usually, materials are rented for a fixed period, about two months. If you will need them longer, as most groups (especially schools) will, then an additional fee is charged. Orchestra parts are normally sent for a shorter period. If your orchestra will need extra rehearsal time, an additional rental fee will be charged. If the show will run over several weekends, then you may need to keep materials for additional time as well—it is hard for the orchestra to play the second week if the parts are returned after the first weekend. Consider all these factors and add up the total rental fees. Add 10 percent for shipping, which you will have to pay in both directions.

For some shows and from some publishers, you must purchase rather than rent materials. In this case, the catalogs will clearly state the cost of such materials. In all other cases, you must write the publisher or agent individually and request a quotation for both royalties and rentals on your production. Most agencies will include a quotation request form in their catalog, and all will also include such a blank form with any perusal copies sent to you. Fill in that form at this time and mail it back.

If you have never done a musical production, be prepared for a shock. Amateur productions of nonmusicals generally pay royalties of $20 to $60 per night. Amateur productions of musicals generally pay royalties of $200 to $500 per night, depending on the show, the size of the auditorium, and the cost of tickets. Rental fees will be in addition to that quotation. It is not at all unusual to be charged considerably more than $1,000 in royalty and rental for a simple three-performance run of a Broadway-generated show. Unknown material and materials written expressly for schools or children's groups will usually be significantly cheaper.

FINAL DECISION

Once you have received quotations for all the shows under final consideration, reexamine and rediscuss the advantages and disadvantages of each script in relation to its now known cost. Make a very simple budget estimate.

1. Consider the royalty and rental fees.
2. Look at the information you supplied when you requested a royalty quotation. Multiply number of tickets predicted by the probable cost of those tickets. That's your estimated income.
3. Subtract royalty and rental fees from estimated income.

What's left is what you will have to produce the show. Given all the expertise available in your committee, does it seem possible that you can actually produce the show well or properly on the remaining money? Examine all the resources at your disposal and considered during Step 6.

If the answer is yes, you've found your show at last. Congratulations! If the answer is yes for more than one of the shows in your final round, then even greater congratulations are in order. If the answer is no, then you *must* find a different show or be prepared for a poor production, financial disaster, or both.

The foregoing process is long and complex and in many ways seems negatively oriented. You start with all kinds of wonderful, exciting ideas and then eliminate them until you are finally left with a single choice. It seems so much more exciting to say, "We really want to do this show," and then to leap into it. But our goal is both to do the show well and to keep our sanity and financial stability while doing so. The only way to do this effectively is to avoid unnecessary problems from the very beginning of the production process. Even in an ideal situation, you will have plenty of necessary problems to occupy your time. Think and consider before you start, so that you may devote your time to necessary problems and not dissipate your talent and time on unsolvable problems that could have been avoided.

If your decision must be approved by an administrator or administrative board, submit your report. Be sure to explain exactly why you decided on this particular recommendation so that they understand exactly what they are agreeing to do.

Step 7: Sign a Contract

The royalty quoted to your group is only an estimate. It will not be considered an agreement until you have signed a contract. Once the organization has agreed to your selection, immediately write to the agency and ask for a contract under the conditions described in your request for royalty information. (In some cases, the royalty quotation will be given on a contract form, so you will not have to make a separate request to see it.)

Do this as soon as possible because conditions do change rapidly. In some cases, royalties may go up, along with inflation, if you wait too long. In others, another group in the area may want to do the same show and preempt the rights.

In response to your letter, you will receive a contract that will state the terms under which you are allowed to produce the show. *Read the contract.* I cannot stress this too much. Every contract is different. When production rights are granted to you, they are granted only under the specific conditions agreed to in the contract. In almost all known cases in which a group has had significant problems with one of the agencies, it has been a result of their not reading the contract before they signed it. The contract will not only say how much you must pay or when you can do the show, but will also include a number of other terms, such as the types or size of credit lines that must be listed in all programs or publicity.

Finally, once you sign the contract, you are committed to the payments scheduled therein. Because the payments must be made in advance, it may be difficult, if not impossible, to cancel the show and hope for any refund.

Now you're ready to begin.

No matter what show you eventually choose, someone in the group is going to complain. There's nothing you can do to prevent this, so don't worry about it. If you have considered the foregoing points, you will satisfy most of the people in the organization. You can never satisfy all of them—don't even try. Now it is time to move on toward the production itself.

3

Conventions of the Musical

Every performance medium operates through a set of conventions—unspoken agreements among the writers, performers, and audience about the way things can or should be done. The musical is, if anything, one of the most conventional performance forms in existence today.

It is unfortunate for the inexperienced producing group that musical scripts use these conventions without explaining either how they work or why they are used. As a result, some parts of the script are confusing or incomprehensible, while the importance of others is often overlooked, leading to disjointed, unsatisfying productions. Thus, before we look at the step-by-step preparation of the show you have just selected, we will briefly examine the most common musical conventions, the problems they can cause for your production if misused, and the problems they can solve if used well.

SCRIPT

The first of the conventions of the musical, unlike other dramatic works, is that its script comes in two separate parts, the libretto and the score. Anyone hoping to stage a musical well must learn to use both parts.

27

Libretto

The libretto contains all the words of the show. It is written in the form of a nonmusical playscript, with some small modifications.

The information in the libretto is given in four parts:

1. dialogue, or words to be spoken
2. song lyrics, or words to be sung
3. stage directions
4. names of characters who speak, sing, or follow these directions

This information is generally arranged in one of two forms.

When the libretto is printed, it usually looks like the page shown in Figure 1. The character name is at the left, usually in capitals. Stage directions are within parentheses and often in italics as well. Dialogue is printed in normal type in paragraph form. Lyrics are printed in verse form, often in capitals as well, to distinguish them clearly from the dialogue. If you purchase materials, this is the form you will probably see.

When scripts are rented, they tend to come in the standard typescript form shown in Figure 2. This form is used in most original productions due to its immediate visual clarity and the large amount of white space it provides in which to make notes during rehearsals. The character name is written in capital letters and centered alone on the line. Stage directions are enclosed in parentheses and usually placed on a line separate from dialogue, indented from the margins for easy recognition. Dialogue is typed as normal text beginning at the left margin. Song lyrics are typed in verse form, usually in capital letters.

Some companies will send you two different versions of the libretto: a director's copy, which contains all of the show's verbal text, and a set of *sides* for each individual character. In a side, the performer receives only the lines he or she will actually say. Compare Figure 3 with the same scene in Figure 2, and you can see how difficult it may be for performers to read or study the side. Sides are a holdover from the years before the invention of the photocopying machine. When copies were made by hand, actors or managers would simply transcribe each actor's role to save time. Only a very few companies still use them, but one of those is Tams–Witmark, which han-

MRS. STONINGTON: They have? Oh, dear!

CHARLIE: Absolutely true. *(pointing at tickets in Gussie's hand)* These are the last ones here.

WOMAN: What will we do?

MRS. STONINGTON: Never fear, ladies. If we can't appeal to the men—which is, after all, no surprise—we will go directly to the lady herself! *(WOMEN cheer)* We will wait for her outside her hotel!

POLICEMAN: Do anything you like, as long as it isn't my beat!

MRS. STONINGTON: Ladies, Onward!

WOMEN *(raising their signs and singing)*:
      WHEN WE FIGHT WE CONQUER VICIOUSNESS AND
        SHAME,
      OUR SHINY TRUMPETS GOING TOOTY-TOOTY.
      ALL GOOD AMERICANS SUPPORT OUR AIM,
      PROTECTING INNOCENCE AND YOUTH AND BEAUTY.
      WE DO OUR DUTY, JUST THE SAME!

(And THEY march off, MEN dispersing afterwards, leaving ROBERT and CHARLIE taking tickets from GUSSIE.)

ROBERT: Awfully nice of you to come up with the money, Gussie.

GUSSIE: What are friends for?

FIGURE 1. Typical libretto format in print (from *The Belle of New York*, by David Grote [unpublished]).

                        MRS. STONINGTON
They have? Oh, dear!

                           CHARLIE
Absolutely true. (pointing at tickets in Gussie's hand)
These are the last ones here.

                            WOMAN
What will we do?

                        MRS. STONINGTON
Never fear, ladies. If we can't appeal to the men -- which
is, after all, no surprise -- we will go directly to the
lady herself!

        (WOMEN cheer)

We will wait for her outside her hotel!

                          POLICEMAN
Do anything you like, as long as it isn't my beat!

                        MRS. STONINGTON
Ladies, Onward!

                           WOMEN
        (THEY raise their signs and sing).

WHEN WE FIGHT WE CONQUER VICIOUSNESS AND SHAME,
OUR SHINY TRUMPETS GOING TOOTY-TOOOTY.
ALL GOOD AMERICANS SUPPORT OUR AIM,
PROTECTING INNOCENCE AND YOUTH AND BEAUTY.
WE DO OUR DUTY, JUST THE SAME!

        (And THEY march off, MEN dispersing afterwards, leaving
        ROBERT and CHARLIE taking tickets from GUSSIE.)

                           ROBERT
Awfully nice of you to come up with the money, Gussie.

                           GUSSIE
What are friends for?

FIGURE 2. Typical libretto format in typescript (same scene as Figure 1).

```
MRS. STONINGTON                                           I/1

   ... has been sold.

                              YOU
   They have? Oh, dear!

   ...What will we do?

                              YOU
   Never fear, ladies. If we can't appeal to the men -- which
   is, after all, no surprise -- we will go directly to the
   lady herself! (WOMEN cheer) We will wait for her outside her
   hotel!

   ... isn't my beat!

                              YOU
   Ladies, Onward!

       (YOU sing with women)

   WHEN WE FIGHT WE CONQUER VICIOUSNESS AND SHAME
   OUR SHINY TRUMPETS GOING TOOTY-TOOTY.
   ALL GOOD AMERICANS SUPPORT OUR AIM,
   PROTECTING INNOCENCE AND YOUTH AND BEAUTY.
   WE DO OUR DUTY, JUST THE SAME!

       (YOU march off)
```

FIGURE 3. Typical libretto format in side (same scene as Figure 1).

dles most of the famous Broadway shows of the fifties and sixties. If you get sides for the cast rather than full librettos, you will need three to five extra rehearsals just so the performers can learn how their lines fit together.

Score

The score provides the musical information about the show. It includes all the music to be performed, with words for the songs and instrumental arrangements indicated.

With most scripts, you receive two kinds of music parts: parts for individual performers and a complete musical score. The performers' parts contain only the melodic line of the songs. The score is used by the conductor to lead the orchestra for the entire show and thus includes far more information about each song as well as many purely orchestral numbers not shown in the performers' music parts.

Most scores for musicals come in the form of a *piano/conductor score*, a peculiar form that manages to be inadequate for all purposes for which it must be used. It reduces the full score to a single piano part, which makes life easy for the rehearsal accompanist but makes it hard for the conductor to know exactly which part of the music each instrument should play. The practical effect on rehearsals is that the conductor must spend the first rehearsal with the orchestra simply trying to find out who actually plays which notes. As a result, the orchestra will almost always need at least one more rehearsal than the conductor would normally schedule.

GENERAL CONVENTIONS

The first and most important convention of all musicals is that they are nonrealistic. This does not mean that they are necessarily pointless or silly, although many are. Nor does it mean that they cannot be serious or concern themselves with genuine problems of human affairs. *Company, Gypsy, A Chorus Line, Carousel, South Pacific,* and *West Side Story* come easily to mind as works that deal with serious issues in a serious manner and need not resort to fairy-tale solutions and one-dimensional or meaningless characterizations. It simply means that musicals by their very nature reject the conventions of realistic stage-craft.

In the mainstream realistic theatrical tradition, the places on stage are designed and constructed to give the appearance of real places. The actors try to reproduce the appearance of real people doing real, everyday kinds of things on that stage within the practical limits set by the need to be seen and heard clearly. Hence, the typical Broadway play of the last sixty years takes place in one room, which is carefully constructed in a three-dimensional setting on the stage.

Musicals are not tied to the conventions and appearances of the realistic theatre. In the "real" world, people do not suddenly burst into song on the sidewalk or dance their way through gang fights or burst into song when a favorite customer appears at the door of the restaurant or sing to their girlfriends about the surrey they want to buy. Once that tie to reality has been broken, the musical is free to change scenes at will, pause for a character to tell the audience how he or she feels, suggest an entire setting with a single prop or a song, or even contain many different places at the same time, none of which would be possible in a realistically oriented production.

A group of musical writers did not get together and say, "A musical must not use realistic stagecraft"; it just happened that way. But this fundamental convention can and should color all understanding of the script. The presence of music and dance frees the script and the production from the requirements of literal realism. The show may emphasize the good or the bad side of life, may deal with serious or shallow problems, may find solutions at its climax that seem to us to fit the nature of the world or not, but no matter what the subject matter, the musical is not ever confined to three-dimensional solid stage-craft.

This knowledge is especially important for school and community groups who have long experience with one-set "realistic" Broadway comedy. The sets in a musical need not be "complete." Since we know that they are nonrealistic, the audience will accept suggestion—you don't have to build all the walls for every set.

At the same time, this convention accepts that characters may sing or dance at any time. Once upon a time, people worried about "justifying" songs in the script, and there were many scenes in operettas in which characters asked, "Would you like to hear a song my mother taught me?" Those days are long gone. In the modern musical, characters simply express themselves in whatever way seems fitting at the time; sometimes that expression is singing, sometimes speaking, and at still other times dancing. They may recognize (as part of their characterization) that they are singing a song, as when Nellie sings "Honey Bun" in *South Pacific*. At other times, they may sing a song and still act as if they were not singing but talking to each other— "Happy Talk" in the same show—or thinking about each other— "Some Enchanted Evening" or "This Nearly Was Mine." Each song has a slightly different purpose in the specific show, so there is no single way to stage the songs.

Like all dramatic works, musicals have plots (except for revues, which by definition have no plot at all). The plot introduces a group of characters, puts them into conflict with each other, complicates the conflict in a variety of ways, and then finally reaches a point at which the conflict is resolved in some way. Musicals, however, tend to have simple plots, in two different ways. First, they are less complex. The plot of most classic musicals can be stated in a single sentence. For example, the plot of *Oklahoma!* is, Can Curly marry Laurey and keep her safe from Jud? Musical plots also tend to be simpler in the structuring of their incidents or the detail with which incidents develop. Compare Thornton Wilder's version of *The Matchmaker* with *Hello, Dolly!*; *Pygmalion* with *My Fair Lady*; *I Am a Camera* with *Cabaret*. The musical versions try to contain the essence of the original work, but always simplify its structure, development, and detail.

This is not because musicals are written for idiots while standard plays are not; it is because musicals have music. Music takes time. A typical, traditional show song has about sixteen lines of lyrics; spoken as poetry, they would take about thirty seconds, but sung they require two or three minutes. This in turn means that things that are clearly stated in nonmusicals must often be hinted at, suggested, or even more often expressed through some common stage convention. In *Romeo and Juliet*, when Romeo first sees Juliet, he embarks on ten lines of gorgeous verse describing the impression she makes on him; when Tony first sees Maria in *West Side Story*, he stares at her and walks toward her as spotlights focus on them both. The musical version may or may not be more effective in performance, but it merely suggests detail and depth rather than actually providing them.

In many musicals the plot will be so simple in both senses that the show must be augmented by a *subplot*. In *Oklahoma!*, for example, there are very few incidents. Curly asks Laurey to marry him; she hesitates, afraid of Jud; Curly warns Jud to leave her alone; she marries Curly; and Jud attacks Curly and is killed accidentally in the fight. To augment the incidents and to provide more humor, the play offers the same plot again with another triangle. Will wants Annie, but he has to overcome the oily attractions of Ali. As Laurey, Curly, and Jud provide the serious romance, Will, Annie, and Ali provide the comic version of the same romantic situation.

The subplot is a holdover from operetta days, when the hero always had a servant who fell in love with the countess's maid at the same time as the tenor courted the soprano, but it is remarkable how persistent the mirror device itself is in even the serious musicals. That is because it serves a most critical function: providing variety. For example, in *West Side Story*, the equivalent of the Tybalt character is changed from a cousin to a brother who also acts as the girl's father, a brother who just happens now to also have a girl in love with him. This adds a subplot mirroring Maria's romantic problems, but more important, it provides a new layer to the musical language of the show, a layer more Latin and more flamboyant than the pure romance of Tony and Maria. In most comedies the subplot carries most of the humor; in more serious shows, the subplot often clarifies the theme and provides the most complex dramatic characters or the most difficult music and/or dance. Thus, you cannot afford to treat such roles lightly in your planning. Whether in a "serious" or a humorous show, the subplot usually involves characters who are more complex, eccentric, or otherwise interesting than the ostensible principal characters. This in turn means that the "supporting" roles often demand far more care and thought in casting than the "starring" roles.

Most people refer to musicals as musical comedies, and thus expect a considerable amount of comedy. There are a number of successful serious shows, such as *Gypsy, Sweeney Todd, Godspell,* or *West Side Story*, but most of these still involve significant comedic elements. Most of the others are comedic both in plot—boy meets girl—and in the attempt to produce a significant number of laughs in the course of the show. Hence, the musical often seems to sidetrack itself with comic routines or situations having little to do with the main dramatic plot of the show and often including comic musical numbers that do not advance the plot in any way. This is sometimes difficult to accept for people trained in conventional theatre and for the more serious musicians who expect everything to make sense, or see such things as sellouts to commercialism. They are not—the musical operates in its own world; it must be taken seriously in the sense that you must stage it sincerely, but it excels precisely because its moods and tones are so mixed. Any attempt to flatten out this mixture will harm the whole show.

STRUCTURAL CONVENTIONS

The musical shares the basic structural elements of nonmusical dramatic works; that is, it generally begins with exposition and builds interest and tension toward a climax. In practice, however, the musical depends on a number of specific, unique structural elements that are not used in any other dramatic form. These elements and devices appear with amazing regularity in almost all successful musicals because they fulfill very important functions.

We will examine these in the order in which they usually appear in the show.

Overture

Before the play begins, the orchestra plays a musical number called the overture (sometimes marked in the score as introduction, prelude, or prologue). This piece has several functions.

The overture signals the audience to quit milling around in the lobby, get into their seats, and stop talking. By occupying four or five minutes, it allows latecomers to take their seats without interrupting the audience's view of the show itself.

It introduces the feeling of the show to the audience, so that they are emotionally prepared for what will follow. This makes it especially important to the production staff, who must find some way to translate that musical feeling into the rest of the production.

Finally, the overture introduces some of the songs that will be heard later in the show. This prepares the audience to recognize the songs when they appear, so that they do not sound quite so new and are thus more pleasant, attractive, and dramatically effective. It also means that the songs will be easier for the audience to remember, which supports their dramatic effect within the show (and, not coincidentally, helps make some songs more popular outside the context of the show itself).

Opening Number

In the traditional musical format, the overture is followed almost immediately by a big musical number involving a large group of people, usually the chorus. This number accomplishes several different things.

First, it gets attention. Thus, it is almost always a big number. In some shows, the opening number tries to set a mood and as a result does not always involve the full cast. *Oklahoma!*, right at the beginning of the modern era, made history by reducing the opening number to its minimum—one voice, unaccompanied, singing, "Oh, What a Beautiful Morning." More intimate shows often follow that lead, as with "Try to Remember" in *The Fantasticks*. But these are rare, and for the most part the opening number will be a big attention-getter.

Most opening numbers are devoted to raw exposition. Not all are as blatant as *The Mikado*'s "If you want to know who we are, we are gentlemen of Japan," but they usually come close. Opening numbers say, "This is where we are, and this is who we are, and this is why we are who, what, and where we are." See the "Train Sequence" and "Iowa Stubborn" that open *The Music Man,* "McConnachy Square" in *Brigadoon*, "Another Openin', Another Show" in *Kiss Me, Kate,* "Willkommen" in *Cabaret*, "Tradition" in *Fiddler On the Roof*, or "Comedy Tonight" in *A Funny Thing Happened on the Way to the Forum*, to name only a handful.

Stars like to have their entrances carefully prepared and generally do not share the stage, so do not expect to find the star in the opening number unless it begins with the star doing a solo ("Tradition" in *Fiddler,* "All That Jazz" in *Chicago,* "Why Can't the English?" in *My Fair Lady,* and so forth).

Although the opening number sounds corny when described, very few musicals have ever successfully dispensed with it. Rodgers and Hammerstein are the most consistently daring: In almost anyone else's hands, *South Pacific* would have opened with "There Is Nothing Like a Dame" rather than the Nellie/Emile scene, or *The King and I* would have opened with either a Siamese Port Song or the children's march rather than with "Whistle a Happy Tune." Yet, despite their success, very few other musical writers have dared dispense with the opening number.

The easiest trap in staging this number is to resort to simple formulas, generally by bringing the chorus on stage in a lump, stringing them out like a choir, and having them sing as loud as possible. All large opening numbers demand volume and energy, but they are not all staged in the same way. The opening number's words tell the audience what to expect; the staging of that number should clearly give the expository information in the song. Being loud and energetic is important, but it is not enough.

Exposition

The events the audience sees depicted on stage consist of two basic types of activities. One activity operates from the present to the future—characters say and do things that demand a response from the other characters involved. This is sometimes called the action. In *My Fair Lady*, Eliza Doolittle asks Henry Higgins to teach her to speak well, and Higgins agrees; Eliza goes to the races and makes a fool of herself; Eliza leaves Higgins because he ignores her, and so on. The other activity operates from the past to the present and merely explains things; this is called exposition.

Normally, exposition explains either events that have occurred in the past or offstage, as when Higgins and Pickering explain events that happened at the embassy ball (during the intermission), or it explains the way a character feels about something. The information in the exposition matters to the play as a whole, as it tells the audience what kind of characters are involved and explains the backgrounds and complications of their situation. But it does not matter in a dramatic sense to the individual characters. This is an important distinction to remember in any stage production and is especially important in musicals. Some of the things to be done on stage demand a response from the other characters, and these things drive the play forward toward its climax. Other things do not demand a response *from the characters*, and as such, although they clarify, amuse, and prepare the audience, they in effect interrupt or slow down the movement of the action.

In most works, the exposition is made at the beginning of the show. The audience must be told who the characters are, what they are like, and where they live so that the audience can understand what they are involved in. In addition, the audience must be given the background of the situation, to understand the conflicts within the plot. If no one explains that Higgins is a speech teacher, that Eliza is a Cockney flower girl, and that Higgins thinks the use of proper speech patterns will enable a person to pass in any class of society, the audience will have no idea what is happening in *My Fair Lady*. Hence, the show begins with several scenes in which this information is given to us in various ways, especially dialogue and the opening number.

As the show progresses, the need for this kind of exposition will fade and the second kind of exposition, explanations of feelings, will predominate. This is the major function of song in the musical.

There is of course dialogue exposition, especially at the beginning of scenes and when related to offstage events. And there are a handful of musical selections that propel the action. But, as a general rule, dialogue drives the action and music provides the exposition.

We can see this more clearly if we examine the music in a classic show such as *My Fair Lady*. Rather daringly, that show dispenses with the big opening number. The gang of Cockneys on the street do not open with a flashy little number explaining how wonderful (or bad) it is to be in London, and so forth. Instead, the show begins with a solo opening number that introduces one of the themes—Higgins's explanation of his theory about language in "Why Can't the English?"

This is followed by:

1. "Wouldn't It Be Loverly," exposition of Eliza's character and dream
2. "With a Little Bit of Luck," exposition of her father's character
3. "I'm an Ordinary Man," exposition of Higgins's character and attitudes to life
4. "Just You Wait," exposition of Eliza's feelings at being bullied by Higgins

There we are, halfway through the first act, and all the songs have been purely expository. This predominance will continue throughout the show; in fact, even in this imaginative, polished, and admirable show, only two songs, "Show Me" and "Without You," are even moderately dramatic in the sense that they demand a response from other characters when they conclude. Not surprisingly, they are also the shortest songs in the show and in general the least famous and least often performed outside the show's context.

The same preponderance of expository songs will be found in almost all musicals. We have looked at this in detail not merely for curiosity's sake but because it has very critical implications for the production staff and performers. Songs stop the action of the play. They are, for the most part, what the audience comes to see and hear, but they do little to "advance" the show. This means that they require considerable effort and imagination in presentation to keep the audience from realizing that the show has in fact stopped for the song.

This is one of the reasons why a song almost never occurs in the middle of a scene. Because a song rarely demands a response from the other characters, it is placed either at a time when the other characters cannot respond—at the end of the scene—or where we will accept exposition that simply prepares us for something else without response—at the very beginning of the scene. Only four of the songs in *My Fair Lady*, for example, do not end their scenes: "You Did It," and "Ascot Gavotte," which are at the beginning and serve as opening exposition; "Why Can't the English?", which is the show's opening number; and "Without You," one of the two "dramatic" songs in the show.

The fact that songs tend to be expository accounts for another peculiarity of most musicals. Most of them have a first act that is almost twice as long as the second, and far more than half the songs occur in the first act. *My Fair Lady* has ten songs in Act I but only six in Act II, an unusually high proportion of new material in the second act. *Cabaret*, for example, has twelve songs in Act I and only three in Act II; *Gypsy* has ten in Act I, four in Act II; and even *West Side Story*, one of the most insistently musical works among the book shows, has only four new songs in Act II, after eight songs and three big dance numbers in Act I. First acts tend to be devoted to exposition because it takes time to prepare all the points of the action so that the audience completely understands the situation. Second acts, once they get under way, tend to be aimed at reaching the climax and can afford fewer pauses or distractions—hence, fewer songs.

The fact that most songs are expository in content establishes a basic attitude for their performance. They are pitched more to the audience than to the characters within the play. Thus, they must be staged toward the audience and not toward the other characters, even when other characters are present. Even when the words of a song are addressed to another character, it does not mean that the performer "sings to" that character; the words of the lyric are intended for another character, but the song itself is for the audience.

Finally, since the songs are almost always expository, the words must be heard clearly. Unless the audience understands every word of every song, they have no understanding of the emotions and background of the characters, and the show has no depth, no matter how flashy the staging may look.

At the same time, it is essential that the production staff for a musical treat the songs as dynamic events. Because the songs are essentially expository does not mean that nothing happens in them; rather it means that whatever happens in them occurs inside the character rather than between one character and another. This means that the song should not be approached as a matter of "staging" or "movement," as happens in so many productions. By this I mean the kind of thinking that says, "We have to vary this, so turn to the right on the first verse, then turn to the left on the second verse, and then sway from side to side on the third." The singers of a musical number, even soloists alone on stage, are not "singers"; they are "characters" expressing their concerns, fears, feelings, tensions, and questions about themselves and about life. The staging problem is how to make those concerns, fears, and so forth visually effective, find some externalization that reinforces what the lyrics and music say, and not simply find something for the performer to do with his or her hands or feet during the song.

Production Number

The production number is one of the most peculiar and most persistent of all musical theatre conventions. When literary oriented critics ridicule the musical as a form it is usually the production number that they focus on first, precisely because the production number is often so nonsensical. But in a very real sense, the production number is what makes a musical a musical, what separates it from a "play with music."

A classic illustration is *Hello, Dolly!* Dolly Levi is a cute but dumpy, middle-aged, barely successful, barely recognized little matchmaker from the suburbs who has decided that it is time she made a match for herself before it is too late. So she arranges for her customer (and her prey) to meet her at the fanciest restaurant in New York City, where she often arranges for couples to meet but where of course she has rarely if ever gone herself. And all of a sudden, she turns into the most famous, sexiest woman in the city, with all the waiters of the restaurant welcoming her in a manner that would be excessive for Princess Di. The song is "Hello, Dolly!," and it is absolutely, intolerably absurd—and absolutely essential.

There is a peculiar but reasonably consistent rhythm to the flow of a musical. At fairly regular intervals, the procession of solos and duets that make up most of the show become somewhat repetitious. Then, for variety and to provide a spurt of interest and enthusiasm, something big, flashy, and energetic must appear, or the show begins to slide down toward failure. The shot in the arm, the change, the burst of razzmatazz that "Hello, Dolly!" provided made the entire show work, gave it the touch of variety and sparkle that the long first act required. The show seems to get its second wind, and the audience seems to shift and settle down for the rest of the act, which is exactly what happens when a production number works well. When this happens, it doesn't matter that the number makes no sense. It works, and so it is in the show.

Production numbers get their name from the fact that a big production is made out of something usually very small or simple. Things are overdeveloped, overblown. More is never enough in a real production number, so dancers, choruses, and the most spectacular sets of the show are usually all thrown in. They also tend to be much longer than any other songs in the show.

In *My Fair Lady*, for example, the first production number, "The Rain in Spain," is imaginatively and unusually small, but it reveals the typical features. It starts with a pointless fragment of dialogue that has simple repetitive lyrics that seem to go on forever

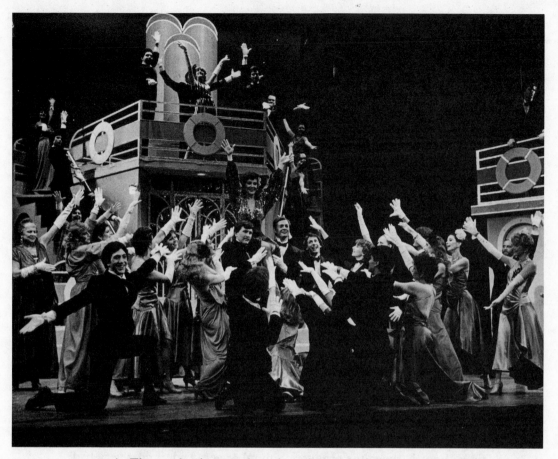

FIGURE 4. The production number. A typical end of number using maximum cast and spectacle. *Anything Goes*, San Jose Civic Light Opera. Directed by C. Michael Traw, scenery by Ken Holamon, costumes by Peter David Heth. Photo by Carl Ballou; photo courtesy San Jose Civic Light Opera.

without any significant variation. Then this little phrase is developed—and developed—until everyone involved is crazed with excitement about what is after all a very simple idea. Except that it is confined to only three people, this is no different from the hysteria and hoopla of "Seventy Six Trombones" in *The Music Man*, "I'm Gonna Wash That Man Right Out of My Hair" in *South Pacific*, "To Life" in *Fiddler on the Roof*, or "A Bushel and a Peck" in *Guys and Dolls*. The more that can be made of less, the better the production number.

Because of their function in establishing and maintaining the energy and variety of the show, production numbers tend to occur at very conventional places in the script. One usually occurs approximately halfway through the first act. If there are two, the second will occur either at the end of Act I or as an opening number for Act II. Occasionally a third occurs in the second act, but this happens in very few shows. This placement holds true even for revues without plots; the placement of these numbers has to do with theatrical pacing rather than plot requirements, so they tend to show up in the same places no matter what shape the rest of the show takes. (The only consistent exception occurs in the operetta, where the production number takes the form of a complex singing number involving both the chorus and the principals, and always comes at the end of an act, particularly when the operetta has more than two acts, as most of them do.)

The production number is a particularly dangerous area in the amateur production. First, it often makes no sense. Second, the script gives little help; because the number as performed in the original production depended on the splendor of the sets and performers rather than the dramatic value of the situation, the script often says something vague like, "they dance until they are exhausted." Third, it depends for its success on precisely those areas that are most awkward for amateur groups—money, spectacle, technical skill—rather than sincerity and talent, which are the strengths of good amateur productions. Fourth, when the production number goes bad, it goes very bad, very quickly. It helps the show as a whole only when it advances or revives audience attention; if it becomes repetitive, it makes the rest of the show seem repetitive and boring, even when it may not be. The production numbers are particular hazards for any production and must be carefully planned to produce the best possible effect (see the discussion on dancing at the end of this chapter). Watch them carefully.

Reprise

As the show progresses, some songs will be sung again, at least in part. When we noted that comparatively few new songs appear in Act II, that did not mean that there is no music. Several songs that were previously sung will be repeated; however, it is important to note that they are not repeated in exactly the same way. When the song appears for a second time, which is called a reprise, it is intended to underscore some important dramatic point. At the end of *West Side Story*, Maria reprises part of "Somewhere" in the scene with Tony's body. This is not to remind us of the song but to restate the emotional difference between the present scene and the first time the song was heard. To hear again the positive dream shared by Tony and Maria as Tony lies dead emphasizes the pain and emotion of the scene, making it in fact more dramatic. This change is often emphasized by having someone else sing the song. When, in *The Music Man*, Harold reprises "Till There Was You," the fact that we first heard it sung by Marian indicates the enormous change in Harold's personality since he fell in love. As the entire company reprises "The Impossible Dream" after Quixote's death in *Man of La Mancha*, we move from sadness to hope and are uplifted, secure that his ideals have not died.

The importance of the reprise is not the repetition but the change that has occurred since the song was first heard. Thus, the reprise must be staged to emphasize that change. One of the most common and effective ways is to stage the reprise to mirror or suggest, without exactly duplicating, the way the song was staged when it was first heard. For example, as Maria sings "Somewhere," she would hold Tony's body to mirror the way he held her when he sang the song originally. In the same way, when Eliza temporarily tries to escape Higgins in *My Fair Lady*, she goes back to Covent Garden and hears the same quartet sing "Wouldn't It Be Loverly," but without her. Thus, to emphasize the fact that she is no longer a part of that world, the quartet might be staged exactly as it was in Act I, Scene 1, to show that she is missing, or it might be staged with various singers taking over her old staging business to show that she is not missed. Either way, her absence would be underlined to show that her emotional situation has changed.

The Show Stopper

In every show there is one special humorous song or production number that provides a special turn for one of the performers. In most cases there is only one of these, which invariably comes in the second act, usually just before the characters are launched into the final sequence of events leading to the climax. In some shows (particularly operettas and more contemporary shows influenced by the operetta pattern), there will be another one about halfway through the first act, sometimes connected to one of the production numbers. These numbers are called *show stoppers* (when they work) because the immediate audience response is so great as to literally stop the show with extended and thunderous applause that prevents the next scene from going on.

Three classic examples are "Brush Up Your Shakespeare" in *Kiss Me, Kate,* "You Gotta Have a Gimmick" in *Gypsy,* and "Officer Krupke" in *West Side Story*; each arrives during a moment of tension, surprises the audience, and provides a sharp burst of humor and pleasure, not quite the same as classical "comic relief" but with much the same effect. There is sometimes a tendency to think these belong to formulaic work, but they appear in even the most sophisticated serious works that meet with any commercial success. Follow *Sweeney Todd* through the degradation, terror, and revenge, and then in Act II just as Sweeney is about to execute his grisly plan up pops "By the Sea"—and in its traditional position, one third of the way through the second act, right where you find "Honey Bun," "Gary, Indiana," "Officer Krupke," "Do You Love Me?," "What Do the Simple Folk Do?," and hundreds of others. The more things change, the more they stay the same, especially in musicals.

The curious and potentially dangerous point about these numbers is that they rarely are performed by the principals. If you have a show like *Fiddler,* for example, in which the star is in almost every song, then don't expect the star to give the show stopper to someone else. But in any other kind of musical, this will go to some small character, often someone never seen again like the strippers in *Gypsy,* or to characters who have no other songs in the show, such as the gangsters who sing "Brush Up Your Shakespeare" in *Kiss Me, Kate.* These numbers can make or break the entire production. When a show stopper doesn't stop the show with laughs and thunderous applause, it will stop it dead in its tracks and kill all the rest of the second act. Not even a dud production number is as dead as a bad show stopper. If the humor doesn't release the tension, if the surprise doesn't surprise and delight, then the number is pointless. Beware here, too, both in casting and in rehearsal. Just because these seem to be "merely" funny songs or belong to unimportant characters, far too many groups pay little attention to their casting. In most cases these numbers will require your most experienced and talented performers because they are often far more difficult than any of the numbers the "stars" of your show will sing.

MUSIC CONVENTIONS

Music conventions are generally noted in the score, but not in the libretto.

Applause Segue

In a regular segue, one piece or section moves directly into the next without pause. In the applause segue, the conductor pauses at the end of a number for audience applause, during which the cast on stage freezes or holds a tableau. Then, as applause begins to die down but before it has stopped completely, the next number begins and the cast goes back into motion.

Bridge

Between most scenes there will be scene changes. As we have noted, these changes are meant to be made as quickly as possible, which is emphasized by a short piece of music called the bridge. The bridge serves two functions: it occupies the audience briefly while nothing is happening on stage (because scenery is being changed), and it signals a change of mood or a continuity of mood between two successive scenes.

   Although they may seem insignificant when you go over the score, bridges are very important to the production. They determine the absolute maximum time available for scenery changes, which in turn limits or controls the kinds of scenery you can use. They also signal important emotional information about the two scenes being bridged, thus indicating the way in which you should stage the scenes on either side of the bridge.

Entr'acte

The *entr'acte* is a second overture, played before the start of the second act. In general, it serves the same functions as the overture: It tells people to put out their cigarettes, finish their drinks, and get back in their seats. In addition, the entr'acte almost always plugs the songs from the show. Even when the overture is very brief or moody, the entr'acte will be snappy and energetic and will reprise the melodies of a number of songs, usually limited to those heard in the first act. This helps to remind people of the songs in case they are to be reprised and, even when not later reprised, may remind the audience of the principal themes or moods of the show.

Play-Off

Singers do not bow or acknowledge applause after each song in the modern musical, but neither do they discourage it by trying to go ahead into dialogue or the next scene. They simply freeze for a moment or two. However, the show then has the problem of getting them going again. This is especially common when a number comes at the beginning of a scene. The solution is the play-off, in which the orchestra repeats part of the song just finished for no reason but to cover the activity while the singers or dancers break from their freeze and leave. When used at the end of a scene, the play-off also serves as a bridge to the next scene.

Underscoring

In some cases, music will be played during dialogue or while action is being performed on stage: This is called underscoring. This occurs in two ways: the introduction of a song may be underscored under dialogue, so that there is a less awkward break in mood between the speaking and the singing; and the emotional intensity of the scene itself may be magnified by music played to accompany it, as we are used to on the soundtracks of television programs and movies.

Given our familiarity with movie underscoring, we might expect it to occur a great deal in musicals. In fact, this second type of underscoring was once quite extensively used in operettas but is very rare in shows written since about 1940. Actors have a distressing tendency to speak at slightly different speeds each evening, with the result that, even with the original casts, the music in the underscoring is not always the same length as the scene it is supposed to accompany. When underscoring is used, it always requires extra rehearsal time to stabilize the timing of the scene.

Vamp

The *vamp* is one of the simplest, most practical, and most common of orchestral conventions. It is a short rhythmic or melodic phrase, usually no more than two measures long, that is repeated ad-lib. It usually appears in the introduction to a number or in the middle during a major change in performers or props. It underscores some stage activity but does not share the problems associated with underscoring, because it can fit any length of time necessary for the stage activity. Once the orchestra begins a vamp, it simply repeats the phrase until it gets the second cue to proceed with the rest of the song. This gives singers and dancers a bit of safety in getting ready to sing or dance and allows each performance a certain amount of flexibility. It can be carried to extremes, of course; all too many of us have heard an orchestra vamp an entire two-minute scene change when the designer had gotten too ambitious or the stage crew too disorganized. But when used well, it is one of the most valuable of all practical devices that appears in the score.

STAGING CONVENTIONS

Most musicals are both long and technically complex. They often require more than a dozen different settings. Even when staged well, they last from two and one-half to three hours, significantly longer than audiences will accept for nonmusicals. But there are still limits on how long an audience will allow a show to run. Thus, the musical demands a method of staging that *moves*, a way to make lots of scene changes without measurably adding to the length of an already long performance.

Because musicals by their very nature are nonrealistic, they have adopted two conventional means of producing this speed, one very old and a second relatively recent.

The rise of the proscenium stage in the seventeenth century introduced a form of painted scenery called the drop, a large, flat, painted piece of material raised and lowered from the space above the stage, where it hung out of view of the audience when it was not in use. The drop dominated European staging until the rise of three-dimensional realism in the late nineteenth century, when most productions adopted the box set, with its three-sided rooms and real furniture. After the various artistic revolutions that came with the twenties, the drop all but disappeared from the legitimate stage.

The musical never surrendered the drop as its fundamental scenic device, because the drop met many important needs more easily than any other type of scenery. First, it provided the maximum scenery in the minimum floor space—a dozen different drops can be stored in four to six feet of stage depth—which is essential for shows that often have a dozen different sets. In addition, those sets could be changed quickly and easily; one or two stagehands pulling up one drop while lowering the next into place could make almost instantaneous scene changes. Also, because drops take no floor space, they leave the floor flat when desired, which is absolutely essential for dancers. Finally, the drop can be adapted to many styles. Before the twenties most drops were realistic in style, following the traditions of realistic oil painters. But after the innovative scenery of the Ballet Russe and the work of the German Expressionists, all the painting styles of modern art could be adapted to stage drops, and were. The painting style then could be used as a device in all the drops to unify the style of the show as a whole, as in the rustically simple yet elegant drops for the original *Oklahoma!* or the Chagall-like drops for *Fiddler on the Roof*.

Although drops look simple, they are both hard to make and hard to use, especially by people who have little experience with them (which includes just about everyone who does not specialize in large-scale musical production). Thus, it may help to examine the drop traditions that date back to the old nineteenth-century melodramas. On a fully equipped proscenium stage, a number of drapery pieces, usually called legs, are hung along the sides to divide the stage from the backstage. These legs block the audience's view of the wings. Drops are hung upstage of these legs, so that when they are lowered into place the legs block off the edges of the drops, hide any puckers, flaps, or frayed edges, and suggest that the scenery continues into the backstage area. There are usually only three or four legs on any stage, so that some of the drops must be hung above leg #1, others above leg #2, and so on. When a drop hung at leg #1 is lowered, it hides all the space behind it. The scenes played in front of the drops at leg #1 came to be called a *scene-in-one* and a scene in front of a drop at leg #2 came to be called *scene-in-two* (see Figure 5).

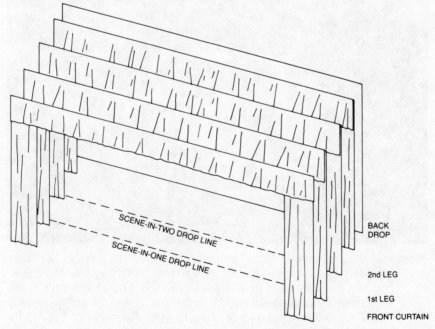

FIGURE 5. Typical proscenium drapery and drop placement

This system allowed the melodrama to move like lightning. While the audience watched a performer in front of the scene-in-one drop, the stage crew made a scenery change behind that drop without interrupting the show. By carefully arranging scenes to alternate between scenes-in-one or scenes-in-two and full-stage scenes, a complex show could be staged without a single break in the on-stage activity.

The musical adopted this system in toto, and almost every successful musical written before 1970 planned its scenes in precisely this manner. Scenes using the full stage are followed by smaller scenes, and vice versa. If you use drops in your production, those drops must be planned and hung so as to work in the same way, with some hung downstage, for scenes-in-one or scenes-in-two, while others are hung to use the full stage space. All props and dance numbers must be planned to fit within the space available either in front of or behind the drop as required.

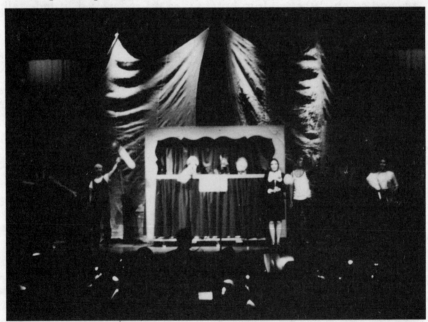

FIGURE 6. Scene-in-one in use. The performers work in front of the front drop (which is cut to resemble circus drapery so that the top of the back drop can be glimpsed behind in photo) while the scene crew is changing scenery behind it out of view. *Carnival*, South High School, Bakersfield, CA. Design, direction, and photo by David Grote.

In the seventies, a new idea began to appear. The one visual problem of the drop show is that all scenes use the full width of the stage, whether using the full depth or simply the scene-in-one. As lighting control improved, this became a drawback rather than an advantage, and directors and designers began to look for ways to use only part of the stage for small scenes. This led to the unit set, in which one basic piece of scenery is on stage for the entire show, with minor changes made to it to suggest different places as needed. This has been a common device of postwar nonmusical theatre and is usually the most common staging solution to Shakespeare's plays in contemporary productions. However, it has until recently seen limited usage outside those areas because changes in the unit are unwieldy. For musicals in particular, the unit limited the amount of spectacular changes possible.

By the early seventies, however, a number of electronic and mechanical innovations made motorized scenery far more flexible and dependable, and a number of shows made use of these devices. The original set for *Company,* for example, consisted of a basic metallic structure with platforms, elevators, projections, and motorized wagons that allowed one basic set piece to stand for six different apartments, several different outdoor settings, and a number of other places as well, often simultaneously. The set for *Dreamgirls* is a group of lighting towers that change position, as if by magic, throughout the show as needed.

In practice, most unit sets will consist of a basic frame and several wagons, which are platforms that carry furniture or props and roll on or off stage as needed. The problem such sets cause for amateurs is that the convention of wagons in the unit, as in *Company* or *Dreamgirls,* only works if the wagons move "as if by magic." When stagehands have to come on stage to move the wagons around, the continuous flow of scenes is interrupted, and the spectacle loses most of its impact.

Whichever convention your script follows, it will rarely be spelled out in detail in the script. For the most part, if the script does not clearly indicate a unit set, it will follow the drop conventions and alternate large scenes with scenes-in-one or scenes-in-two. Without an awareness of these conventions, the entire production could be seriously harmed. Not too long ago, I visited a production of *My Fair Lady* that ran more than four hours; no one forgot their lines and no

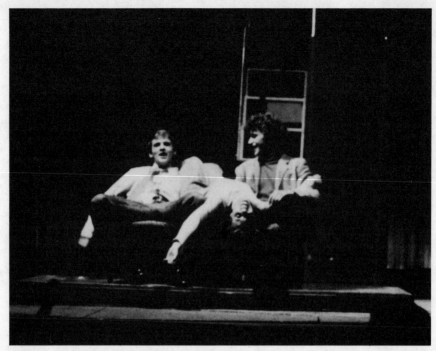

FIGURE 7. Unit set. A wagon within a simple unit set, allowing changes of
scene by rolling on differing furniture props in front of scaffold-
ing that is a permanent set piece. *Company*. South High School,
Bakersfield, CA. Design, direction, and photo by David Grote.

scenes were added—the principal problem was that the drops for the
scenes-in-one were hung too far upstage. Thus, whenever the performers left Higgins's study, the audience had to wait while the stagehands manually moved all the furniture off and then lowered the drop
for Doolittle's or Freddy's street scenes, and then wait again while they
manually moved all the furniture back on for Higgins's study. This
alone added almost thirty extra minutes of running time to the first
act, in turn forcing an extra intermission that only further extended
the show.

It is important to stress that this does not mean you must always
do the show the way it was done in New York. Some drop shows can
be adapted to units, and some units can be adapted to drops, and both
can be done more simply than in their New York version. It does mean
that, when you start making adjustments to fit your own stage and
budget, you must make those adjustments within the unspoken as-
sumptions of musical staging, or they will not work.

DANCING CONVENTIONS

In almost all scripts, the dance directions will be: "They dance." This is not much help to either the choreographer or the stage director. The dancers must find their guidelines between the lines of the libretto and in the music of the score. Musical scripts will provide almost no specific, and very little implicit, information for anyone about the dance to be used in the production. This is not because dance is unimportant; in some cases it will be the single most critical factor separating a good show from a poor one. Rather, it is simply a result of the fact that no one has found a simple, efficient way to write down a dance. But don't be misled by the apparent brevity of the dance in the script—it is always important to the show and difficult to develop.

(The videocassette may change all this. It is now possible for a licensing agency to provide a tape of the original choreography of a show and, for an additional royalty fee, license you to duplicate it in your production. Although no one has done so yet, the possibility exists, and choreographers may soon take advantage of it in order to increase their share of the royalty for amateur productions.)

Just as the musical has its own unique approach to staging, so too does it have a unique approach to dance. Musical comedy dance has traditionally been aimed at an audience that for the most part has feared or disliked ballet and any other forms of "artsy" dance. As show songs are popular music, so also is show dancing popular dance. As such, it is based on the traditions of popular dance performed by people listening to popular music, first in folk materials and then later in the dance halls and ballrooms of American cities. Although choreographers consistently borrow from the vocabulary of both the ballet and the many variations of modern dance, the basic core of all musical comedy dance is ballroom dance "writ large." It is far from the world of the trained dancer, which is of course the principal reason why amateurs, with stamina and good coaching, can do it well.

Thus, the choreographer for a musical faces two different, contradictory problems. First, the seriously trained dancer cannot usually use that training—even if there are enough dancers available in your group, the traditions of the musical are different. People who try to force classical work into the show invariably fail unless they modify it severely.

At the opposite pole, people who simply try to use popular dance steps usually fail even more completely. Popular dance is based on participation, not observation. When we waltz or foxtrot or join a folkdance, we take our pleasure from the repetition of a few simple steps. When we watch other people repeat the same simple steps over and over we feel like the kids lined up against the wall at the high school dance, watching everyone else have fun while we're too afraid or too ugly to participate. Thus, although the dancers in a musical comedy may waltz, they cannot simply duplicate waltz steps for three minutes; they must do something more with them.

Although *On Your Toes, Oklahoma!*, and *Carousel* employed the techniques of classical ballet in the musical, these techniques were still, for the most part, confined to the narrative elements, usually in "dream" sequences. Modern dance followed the same path, as in the "rumble" in *West Side Story*. Production numbers continue to be built on the basics of popular dance. As first Latin American and then Black influences were felt in the ballroom, they became acceptable on stage, so that now the show choreographer has access to an eclectic vocabulary that includes steps, lots of hip movement, athleticism, and full-bodied posturing borrowed from the disco floor. Aerobics and various forms of street dancing continue to expand the vocabulary that is both familiar to the performers and acceptable to audiences, although these are sometimes difficult to adapt to the musical tone of most of the classic musicals. But the core of this vocabulary is still the dance floor, not the dance studio. It is from the dance floor that almost all musical comedy dance numbers must be built.

One of the traditional solutions for a successful dance number in the musical is to add more bodies. If we watch one person do a tap dance that consists of a basic time step and two variations, we get bored quickly. For some inexplicable reason, if we watch the same step being done by twenty people, we will watch for minutes at a time and often cheer at the finish. One person kicking is okay for a quick effect, but the entire cast lined up for high kicks like the Rockettes will stop even the most sophisticated show (as in the finale of *A Chorus Line*). When the budget allows, these extra bodies are often accompanied by gaudy spectacle. The old revues of Ziegfeld and Carroll staged huge production numbers that involved little more than girls wearing outrageous costumes walking among flamboyant scenery, a tradition continued by Las Vegas casino shows, but the same impulse lies behind such numbers as the "March of the Siamese Children" in

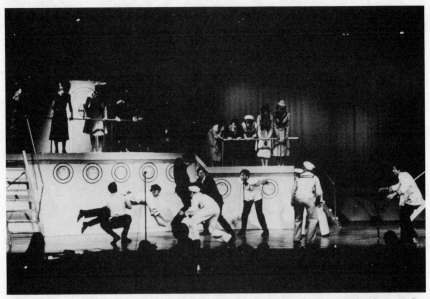

FIGURE 8. Nondancing Dance. Narrative mimetic elements substituted for part of dance number. *Anything Goes*, South High School, Bakersfield, CA. Choreography by L. Michael McQuerrey, design, direction, and photo by David Grote.

The King and I, the joust scene in *Camelot*, or the first act finale of *Sunday in the Park with George*.

Another approach is to build part of the dance around props or costume pieces. Top-hat-and-cane numbers are the most obvious and traditional examples, but the opportunities are almost limitless, depending on the show and the props available.

A third approach, when the number of trained dancers is limited, is to give more dances to soloists or small groups who can do more complex material than the large group. This must be used sparingly, so that the audience does not catch on that you are hiding limited skills, but it provides a way to do far more complex dances than would otherwise be possible.

A fourth approach, more practical for amateurs with limited budgets and skills, is to concentrate on the narrative elements in the dance number. The dance serves a function in the plot, however minimal; underline that function by giving the dance a little story, which allows you to mix mimetic elements with the dance. This establishes some visual variety and builds each number to an ending without resort to either overwhelming expense or the need for well-trained dancers.

57

4

Budget

Once a script has been selected for production, the next practical step is preparing the production budget, which includes all the financial planning for all aspects of the production.

The most important point to remember about the budget is that there is no point in making one unless there is some hope that you can stay within it. No budget should be a straitjacket, for you will always need to make adjustments as the production develops—extra tickets may be sold, the bid on paint from the supplier may change, the person who agreed to lend the sofa will change her mind so that you will have to rent one, and so forth—but the budget should reflect realistic expectations about all money involved in the show.

In some senses, the budgeting process is another of the many chicken-and-egg propositions associated with musical production: You cannot project an accurate budget until you have carefully analyzed all the physical requirements of the script and developed designs, and you cannot make practical designs until you know the budgetary limitations within which the designers must work. For this reason, the production staff should make the analysis of the detailed script requirements described in Chapter 5 simultaneously with the budgeting process discussed here. Then, their analysis and input must be a significant factor in the way funds are allotted in the final budget.

PREPARING THE BUDGET

There are two basic approaches to budget planning. One is to consider what an ideal production would cost and then commit yourself to finding sufficient income to cover that cost. This is ideal, but dangerous. It is generally the way an original New York production is developed, and like a New York production, it puts the financing group at great risk if ticket sales do not in fact come in as hoped. You will not face financial risks of the same magnitude as those faced in New York—many New York expenses, such as professional, union-scale salaries, theatre rental fees, or major media advertising campaigns will not appear in your budget. But then neither will you be able to charge $40 or more per ticket for eight shows each week for several years to cover those expenses. In particular, if you commit yourself to full-scale scenery, costuming, and special effects, you could come very close to matching the New York figures for those items and could easily spend hundreds of thousands of dollars.

The second approach is to consider the probable income and then find a way to make the best possible production within that limit. This is more difficult in many ways because it demands a great deal of care and imagination. When done without imagination, it produces cheap, amateurish productions. All things considered, however, it is by far the best way to approach the budget in most organizations. As long as the production staff agrees that it is possible to produce the show effectively for the money available, then this budget approach provides a practical and financially sound foundation for planning the rest of the production.

If this is your first production or the first musical production in some time in your community, then either approach will have its problems. Without some past experience in the local situation, it is extremely difficult to make any valid estimates of income. In such a situation, always be conservative.

A practical budget should consider each of the following areas.

Income

Ticket sales

Ticket sales cover money received from all admissions to see the production. In some states, ticket sales must be called "donations" in order to maintain the nonprofit status of the organization, but whether charged or donated, this is the fee a person pays to occupy a seat and watch the show.

For some groups, ticket sales can be predicted with reasonable accuracy. In high schools, for example, the musical tends to draw far larger crowds than other nonmusical dramatic productions. In my experience, this is a factor more closely related to cast size than to the nature of the material selected itself. For nonmusicals, most of the schools I have known have drawn fifteen to twenty people per cast member. For musicals, the ratio changed to thirty to forty people per cast member. Because the musical almost always has much larger casts, that translated into audiences four or five times larger than for nonmusicals. For some schools, particularly those in small towns in the Midwest and South where there is only one high school, the formula is higher; for big city schools in parts of town with little sense of community, the formula is lower. For schools below the high-school level, the audience is usually confined to only family and immediate friends of the cast.

In colleges, the size of the audience depends on the nature of the campus and its relations with the community. In small schools with a large percentage of students who live on or near campus, attendance will usually be about twenty to thirty people per cast member. In large colleges or in colleges with big commuter populations, the attendance depends almost completely on community relations and advertising and is much closer to the typical problems faced by community theatre groups.

Community theatre attendance is much harder to predict. For such groups, ticket sales are closely tied to the impression the group makes within the community. The base for that audience will usually be from thirty to forty people per cast member, just as in a school, but the reputation of the organization, the size and appearance of the building, the recognizability of the show, and the nature of the advertising campaign will eventually determine whether or not sales exceed that figure and by how much.

Actual income from ticket sales is a matter of number of tickets multiplied by the price paid for those tickets.

However, the price of the tickets may have a significant effect on the number of tickets sold. If prices are too high, people will not buy them. But if prices are too low people will assume that the show is not worth anything and will not buy them either. Finding a successful middle ground is always difficult. In general, people expect the price of a ticket for a professional production to be comparable to that of a reasonably good restaurant dinner, and they in turn expect an amateur production to cost less than such a good dinner would cost in the local community. Another good parallel is the local first-run movie theatre; most community theatre groups can charge adults $1 to $3 more than for a movie ticket without driving away potential customers and should never charge less than a movie ticket would cost. Schools usually find that the price of a movie ticket is their maximum.

In most situations you will wish to have different prices for some groups. Student and senior citizen tickets are generally discounted, for example. If you use reserved seating (see the section on tickets further on in this chapter), this will mean offering tickets at several different prices. If you do decide to use reserved seating, you can generally expect that the most expensive tickets will sell much better than the cheaper ones for reasons that defy rational explanation.

Donations

Few organizations can expect to finance the musical completely by the sale of tickets. Donations of some kind are almost always essential.

Many donations are in cash, particularly if the production is done by an ongoing organization. Local businesses often make donations to arts organizations as part of their effort to improve their public image and provide deductions on their tax forms. Community theatres find such cash donations invaluable.

Many other people and companies will donate goods or services that can provide as much help to the budget as cash donations. Props and costume items may be borrowed from individuals or groups, tickets may be printed free by a local company in return for a small advertising blurb (soft drink companies in particular like to do this), room and board for a visiting choreographer may be offered by someone, and so on. All such donations should figure in your budget, if they can be predicted with any accuracy.

Concessions

For many groups, the extra bit brought in by concession sales at intermission is often the difference between profit and loss on any show. Although the profit from concessions will usually be small in comparison to ticket sales, the fact that it is profit makes it extremely important to the overall budget. Having been trained in movie theatres, which are supported by their concessions rather than their tickets, people are generally willing to buy overpriced drinks during intermissions; if you have a large crowd, and especially if you have a large crowd of children and young adults, this can add up to a significant figure. If the probable audience is primarily adult, the income will be less, unless you are one of those rare groups in states that allow you a license to sell wine and beer at intermission.

These three sources constitute the income you may expect for the production.

Expenses

Royalties and rental of parts

The figure for royalties and rental of parts is quoted when you sign your contract for the show and is a fixed amount, no matter how you adjust your other figures (see Chapter 2). Remember, however, if during the budgeting process you decide to change ticket prices or the building in which you perform, royalty must be renegotiated. Likewise, the rental fees may vary slightly depending on how many additional copies of parts you finally decide to order.

Facility

This item covers all the expenses associated with the building in which you will perform the show. In most cases, you should be able to predict this accurately.

If you rent a facility, expenses in this area will include the following:

- Rental of stage
- Security deposits, which should be refundable
- Utilities, if figured separately
- Staff, if a Technical Director or paid stage crew is required as a part of the rental agreement
- Rental of rehearsal space
- Rental of storage space
- Extra janitorial services unless included in rent

If you have access to a rent-free facility or own your facility as a school or community theatre usually does, then this figure will be quite small or even nonexistent. For all other groups, this will often be the largest expense, exceeding even the cost of royalties or orchestra. If there is an area in which you need to concentrate energy looking for donations, this has the highest priority.

Salaries

If you hire professional staff, they must of course be paid. The amount actually paid will vary enormously depending on the local situation, the size of the production, and the availability of such professionals. If they come from out of town, their salaries will reflect the need for room and board while they stay.

Even when the staff is voluntary, many of the creative staff will expect an honorarium. Although there are legal differences between the two, the practical difference between an honorarium and a salary is that the salary pays the worker, and the honorarium pays the worker's babysitter. Honorariums are usually paid to each of the three directors, the rehearsal accompanist, and to designers if the sets or costumes are actually designed rather than rented. Although rarely paid, honorariums should also be offered to the stage manager and to anyone else who is expected to be at almost all rehearsals or to devote a significant amount of time and creative, skilled effort and who will have no opportunity to receive applause on stage. Some will refuse, others will be grateful for anything, no matter how small; in most cases, it is the thought that counts. But these can add up to several thousand dollars for community groups.

In schools, most of the staff will be either teachers or students who are already paid in some way (salary or grades) for their work. There, honorariums and/or salary usually are limited to the accompanist and any staff member who must be brought in from outside the school. These can generally be estimated in the lower hundreds.

Publicity

Publicity includes the cost for all posters, programs, handbills, photos used in publicity releases, advertising graphics, and advertising space or time. If you want to, you can spend more on publicity than on the production itself. The publicity costs for many professional shows approach that figure. But, in general, there are limits to what can and should be spent, and there is no reason to spend an inordinate amount of money on publicity.

The key to a successful publicity campaign is to spend only enough money on publicity to reach the audience you want or seriously expect to come to your production.

Thus, the first step in planning the publicity budget is to make a realistic estimate not only of the size of the potential audience but also the composition of that audience. In many cases, groups tend to spend publicity money extravagantly for a return that does not exist. For example, only high schools in small communities with a single school can realistically expect to draw people from the community at large. The overwhelming majority of a school audience is made up of other students, parents, relatives, and immediate neighbors of the people in the cast. In the same way, the audience for a production sponsored by a community charity is composed primarily of people who know the cast, care about the charity, or know the people involved in the charity. Only groups with already well-established musical traditions and reputations can expect to draw significantly beyond their basic audience group.

Once you have determined what group you can most effectively attract, publicity should be planned to reach them. There is little point in taking out newspaper ads, for example, for shows at the high school, because students rarely read the newspaper. But radio spots on the rock station just might be effective, even when the show is not rock oriented, because students listen intensely to that medium.

There are hundreds of ways to publicize a production and hundreds of variations depending on the community in which you live, the policies of various media in the area, and the amount of money you have available. Some of the works listed in the Selected Bibliography will provide additional help and ideas.

Finally, remember to examine your contract in planning and budgeting all publicity campaigns. Most contracts will include specific provisions that apply to publicity. In particular, they will indicate a number of names from the original production that must be given credit in any posters, ads, or articles. In some other cases, they will put specific limits on the kinds of advertising that may be used. Tams-Witmark, for example, does not own rights to the Peanuts characters, so their contract for *You're a Good Man, Charlie Brown* specifically forbids use of the cartoon figures in advertising. Many groups try to use the advertising logo from the cast album or the New York publicity, which increasingly is separately copyrighted and requires additional fees for legal use. Read your contract, and stay within the terms specified in that contract.

Tickets

Budgeting tickets requires more than merely asking a printer what a set of tickets would cost. After the production itself, the most meaningful contact the audience has with your organization is through ticket sales. Hence, a successfully planned and organized ticket sale serves as publicity and public relations for the show as a whole, as well as providing the means to receive and account for funds.

The primary budgeting question is the choice between reserved and unreserved seating. Unreserved seating is simpler and cheaper than reserved seating, because there is only one kind of ticket that must be printed, and such tickets can be sold by anyone at any time. Reserved seating costs more because each ticket must in effect be printed separately and sold separately, but it can often result in better ticket sales. Which type of seating you use depends on the audience and the theatre in which you perform.

In unreserved seating, the ticket gives admission to the building, and seats go on a first-come, first-served basis. This is favored by younger and more informal audiences who don't like to be confined to a specific place. Unreserved seating also allows you to sell tickets at different prices to different audiences: You can offer different prices to students, to seniors, to children, or to any other discount group. As long as the money received matches the number of the various types of tickets collected, the accounting is simple. In general, the sales are simple as well. Cast and crew members can be sent out in the community to sell tickets on their own, which is an effective publicity campaign, particularly among school groups. Anyone can buy a ticket from any person at any time and still get as good a seat as anyone else at the performance. The only danger here is that most groups overprint tickets, knowing that many of the sellers will not sell all their tickets. But occasionally they do, so that more people show up for shows than there are seats for them to sit in.

Reserved tickets are more complex. The ticket guarantees the holder a specific seat. This is favored by more mature audiences, who like to know what they are getting before they arrive and who like to believe that they can linger over dinner for a few minutes and still have a good seat even though they arrive only a minute or two before (or after) the show starts. Reserved seating is especially effective in large or awkwardly shaped theatres, where some seats are clearly better than others. In addition, the fact that seats are reserved suggests that the seats might in fact all be gone if the buyer doesn't get one right away, which encourages advance sales and better attendance. Finally, reserved seats can often be sold for more than unreserved seats; there is an important psychological factor in having other people know you have bought the "best," and people who will pay to get a good seat will often not buy any ticket at all if they can't buy the most expensive one.

But reserved seats also have disadvantages. First, they must be sold from a central location, either in person or by phone. This requires a stable, regular ticket-sales staff, available for long time periods, which often requires additional expense for telephone lines and even salaries. Reserved seats also make it extremely difficult to offer discounts to various groups; the accounting is so complex that it is beyond the ability of most organizations, even professional groups. You will also have to make some hard policy decisions about telephone reservations, many of which can backfire when customers don't understand the policy correctly and thus can give the organization an unfavorable public image.

Tickets can be printed very cheaply at the local level, as long as there are no reserved seats and there is careful control of the number of seats sold. If you wish to use reserved seating, local printers can usually provide the service, as well as a number of national companies that specialize in computer-generated tickets.

Scenery, costumes, and props

The expenses for scenery, costumes, and props are significant. They are lumped together here because they are so closely interrelated. The precise cost for each of these items will depend on the nature of the specific requirements of the script; the size, shape, and equipment of your facility; the nature of the specific designs made to meet those requirements, and whether such items are constructed locally or rented.

The best way to estimate the cost for budgeting purposes is to contact several of the companies who rent scenery and/or costumes for musicals. Ask them for their basic rental prices or, if they rent "complete shows," the basic rental fees for such packages. If you decide to design and build yourself, the cost should not exceed the cost of the rental. (See page 74, Rental *vs.* Construction, for the advantages and disadvantages of rentals.)

Light and sound

Expenses in this area are quite variable, depending on the facility used. When you rent or borrow a stage it will have some lighting and sound equipment. This is usually inadequate for what you need to do a musical. Unless the stage is remarkable, you will need to rent or borrow additional lighting equipment (follow-spots in particular, as well as other instruments or dimmers) and some sound equipment (microphones in particular). Be sure to determine exactly what equipment is available and included when you rent the stage. Then, confer with your electronics staff to determine exactly how much additional equipment is needed. Some of this will be available from local sources, but others must be rented from theatrical suppliers.

Even if all else is on hand, you will have to buy color media for the lighting instruments.

Orchestra

One of the most complex decisions you must make is whether or not to use a full orchestra. A discussion of the possibilities for varying the orchestration follows in Chapter 5. Any decision in this area costs money, from the rental of orchestral parts or instruments to the payment of the musicians. Do not finalize the budget plans until you have discussed the situation with the music director in detail. If the orchestra must be augmented, instruments substituted, or eliminated in favor of a piano combo, be sure that is completely understood before setting the budget. Many organizations have seen their potential profits disappear during dress-rehearsal week when they suddenly had to pay fifteen union-scale musicians more than the cost of all the scenery and costumes.

Makeup

Most groups forget to allow for cost of makeup, but in amateur productions, the organization usually needs to provide the basic makeup supplies for the entire cast. For a first show, this will cost several hundred dollars, because you must also provide the basic application equipment such as sponges, brushes, mirrors, and so on. However, once the basic equipment is on hand, makeup supplies will generally last through several shows and, except for specialty items, will be a minimal expense (under $100) for most succeeding productions.

Shipping

Shipping is the sneakiest item in the budget and traditionally the one that ends up turning a profit back into a loss. Any items from outside the local community, whether purchased or rented, will involve shipping charges. For rented items, charges will apply in both directions—for receipt and return. Such charges are in addition to regular quoted costs and are always paid by the organization receiving the shipment. For large items, items shipped long distances, or items shipped by express-service methods, this cost can be significant. In most cases, 5 percent of any purchase or rental prices is a conservative estimate. Be sure to include at least that much in your budget for everything from scripts to scenery to makeup supplies—anything that requires shipping to or from an out-of-town supplier.

Programs or playbills

Each member of the audience expects to receive a program containing information about the show and identifying the performers. Programs cost money, but how much depends on what else the organization wants to do with the program.

Many groups, in an attempt to signal that the production is important or of "professional" quality, print very extensive and expensive programs—like the ones they receive at the symphony or the big-city professional theatre production. In turn, they finance these programs by selling ads to local merchants. The only problem with this comes when the tail starts wagging the dog: So much effort and money must be expended to put the program together, to see printers and sell ad space and make layout that the production itself is slighted. In addition, if ad sales aren't up to expectations, production funds must be siphoned off to cover the program printing costs.

In my own experience there is a limit to the power of the playbill. A glossy playbill does no more than put the audience in a receptive mood; it does not affect the quality of the show. If you must make a choice between money and time for the production or for the playbill, the show itself is far more important.

Whatever method you choose for printing your programs, there is only one critical factor: *Get the information right.* Nothing destroys a performer like having a name misspelled in the program. In the same way, no matter how glossy the program may be, if it is riddled with typos or factual errors, the organization will look like a group of illiterates or ill-informed provincials. Accuracy and completeness are more important in the long run than glossy paper and photos.

General business expense

An allowance for general business expense is often overlooked in most budgets. Daily operation of the organization and the production usually requires some office expense. Depending on the organization, this will include the following items:

- Postage
- Stationery and office supplies
- Checking account fees
- Interest
- Copies and duplication of contracts, information sheets, publicity releases, schedules, and the like
- Purchase order or billing forms
- Incorporation fees
- Business licenses
- Telephone installation and/or charges
- Answering machines, services, and so forth
- Taxes

BALANCING THE BUDGET

Developing a budget requires the balancing of interests among all these areas. Once the show has been selected and the contract signed, some of the expenses are predetermined and fixed. These include the royalty payment, rental fees for the scripts and parts, and the rent for your facility. No matter what else you decide, these figures stay the same. But all other parts of the budget are open to discussion and variation. What you spend on scenery, publicity, tickets, and other such areas of the production depends primarily on what you wish to accomplish in each of those areas. You may spend as much as the original producers spent, or practically nothing.

This is a serious question because, in a very real sense, money is part of the point of the musical. The audience expects to see spectacle when they come to see a show; they want attractive scenery and many interesting costumes, and they want to hear a good orchestra. They do not necessarily want *only* those things, but they are part of what is commonly associated with the very word *musical*. More money will not automatically make a show more successful, but less money will very often hurt it. In any rational budget, however, the goal is not to spend every cent you can find (which sometimes seems to be the goal in Broadway productions) but to spend every cent that you have effectively. Draw up the budget so that you can get the absolute maximum effect from the minimum amount of money.

To do this, the organization must be willing to balance interests. Is it better to spend the extra money to obtain competent orchestra players than to pay for advertising spots? Does the security given audience members by reserved seating justify the extra expense of reserved tickets and a central box office to sell them? Can a scenic effect be produced simply and more money concentrated on spectacular costuming, or should money be concentrated on scenery while costumes are simplified? Should programs be mimeographed rather than printed in order to have more money for extra microphones? Hundreds of similar questions must be considered before a budget can be proposed with any accuracy.

No one can predict how each show must be balanced, but hard experience has given me the following principles:

1. If you have the money, spend it. Fancy sets and costumes put audiences for amateur productions in a receptive mood and encourage them to overlook minor performing lapses.
2. The audience will accept simple scenery if it is well constructed and the performers are good. If the cast is not good or the scenery looks tacky rather than simple, the simplicity of the production will become a negative factor.
3. If you have limited funds, costumes come first, before scenery, for two reasons: a) costumes can act as a form of scenery if well designed, while scenery cannot act as costumes no matter how well designed, and b) costumes are on the actors, whom (one hopes) the audience will be watching more often than the scenery around them.
4. Money spent should always be spent visibly. With only a handful of exceptions, there is no such thing as "wretched excess" in musical production. Do things as cheaply as possible, but be sure that they always look as expensive as possible.

Budget Crises

There are occasional budget crises when ticket sales and donations do not come in as predicted. But far more often crises arise because the group has not accurately predicted expenses. Unless you prepare the budget carefully and thoughtfully, you will have continual monetary and personal problems throughout the entire production.

The critical factor in making budget decisions is that it must be done with adequate information. You cannot simply set aside $50 or $500 or $5,000 for a particular item and expect it to be adequate. Check with potential suppliers for estimates, discuss options *in detail* with the members of the production staff who are likely to know costs and problems in a particular area, and collect as much information as possible before trying to balance the interests of each aspect of the production.

The budget must balance on paper. This will not guarantee that it will still be in balance when the show closes, for some ticket sales may not happen, some emergency may force a cost overrun in advertising or scenery, or the pianist may break an arm, forcing you to hire another, more expensive musician. Any number of other problems may arise that demand unforeseen expenditures, but there is no hope of the budget balancing at the end if you cannot balance it at the beginning. Be absolutely realistic about all your estimates; do not try to pretend that you can construct the costumes for *Gypsy* for $500 when the designer, the director, and the costume rental house all say that's impossible. At the same time do not pretend that you will be able to spend $5,000 on those costumes when you know that you are likely to sell only $6,000 worth of tickets for the entire show.

Although budget balancing seems a purely monetary issue, momentary crises can quickly turn it into an extremely destructive emotional issue in any organization. Every person in the production is affected by decisions made about the use of the money available. If all their interests are not balanced fairly, the resulting disagreements can grow so intense that they can lead to the collapse of any production, even when sufficient money for a good production is available. Of all the crises in musical production, these are the most common; yet they are also the most easily preventable.

Such crises tend to arise for a simple reason: The production staff is committed to producing the best show they know how to produce while the administration or board of directors of the organization must of necessity be committed first to the financial solvency of the organization as a whole. Those two positions are often in conflict. Production staff will have ideas that require more money; administrative staff will consistently demand that less money be spent; the production staff will complain about the ignorance of the administrative staff, and the administrative staff will complain about the profligacy and irresponsibility of the production staff. Complaints will escalate into conflicts until the show suffers.

These conflicts can be prevented in only one way: the production staff must be involved in the formation of the budget. In almost all established organizations with which I have been associated or have observed, the administrative staff picks the show, establishes the budget, and only then looks for the production staff. In such cases budgets rarely take into account the specific nature of each individual musical.

As an illustration, a community theatre once offered me a job directing *Gypsy*. When I asked what the budget would be, they told me I would have $500 for everything after royalties and salaries. Anyone who has examined the script for *Gypsy* knows that you could spend that much on Gypsy's clothes alone, without even considering the fifty-odd other characters and seventeen sets. No one on that particular board had considered what such a show might cost from the viewpoint of actual production. They just "always" budgeted $500 for production of shows. They also *always* had fights with directors and designers who *always* went over budget. Somehow they had never connected the two things.

Such problems could have been easily prevented if that particular board had asked anyone who knew something about production costs what the particular show they had chosen was likely to cost and then listened to such people when they explained. There will always be problems with money, even with the best prepared budgets, because there will always be emergencies and unforeseeable problems, but if you try to prepare a budget without input from the production staff, you can always expect continual budget crises and bad feelings during rehearsals.

For schools there is an additional kicker in the budget process. In many schools the budget will be entirely dependent on ticket sales. In many others, however, some or all of the budget will come from funds provided by the school. It is absolutely essential that you spend *all* of that money, whether you need to do so or not. Governmental agencies, including schools, operate on a peculiar theory that says, "If you don't overrun your budget, then obviously you don't really need the money." There is no reward for saving a few dollars. In fact, if you find a good deal on scenery materials and come in $400 under budget on a show, you can be guaranteed that your budget for the next one will be reduced by $400 or more. In most places you would expect that when you overrun your budget it would be taken as proof of poor management and punished in some fashion; in schools, it is usually rewarded with additional funds in succeeding years. This is absurd, but it is a widespread practice. If you squeeze any money at all out of your principal, see that it is not only budgeted but that it is also spent.

Finally, remember that the bulk of expenses must be met in advance. Most agencies will not ship any scripts or music parts until royalty and rental fees have been paid in full. Unlike nonmusicals where royalties are due a week or so before opening, you cannot wait for advance ticket sales to give you the money to pay this. Somewhere along the line you must have saved, budgeted, or borrowed the money to pay this enormous fee several months before the show opens and usually a month or so before you begin ticket sales.

Rental vs. construction

In many cases construction of scenery, costumes, or both for a musical production is far too complex for most organizations to handle. As a result many groups turn to rentals, which have a significant effect on the budget for the show.

There are some obvious advantages to renting much or all of the show. Not the least of these is that it eliminates most of the need for local labor backstage, where it is always difficult to find good people. In addition you get material that at least promises to be of professional quality, although this will vary depending on the companies you choose to rent from. I know of high schools that have been able to rent the same drops and costumes used in the New York production of a show, which provides a kind of quality and spectacle that the local group could never hope to reproduce even if they had the funds available to try.

Even when you want to design and build most of the show yourself, there are always problem areas that you cannot solve. As a result there are a number of companies across the country that will rent almost anything needed for a particular musical show. In the case of the most popular shows, many companies will rent complete packages, so that you can simply order the show as a single set of scenery pieces, costumes, or both.

There are a few drawbacks to rentals, however. The most obvious one is that you cannot keep the material for future use. If you construct a drop for *South Pacific*, when the show is over you can repaint it and use it again for *My Fair Lady*; the only additional cost is new paint. If you rent a drop for *South Pacific*, when the show is over you send it back; then for *My Fair Lady* you pay the full cost of a new rental. It should be noted, however, that most musical sets and costumes cannot in fact be reused. Only one show in the world looks like *Li'l Abner*, only one popular musical is set on a South Sea island during World War II, and so on. When you construct your own scenery, costumes, or props, they can usually be reused only by reducing them to their raw materials again. Drops can be completely repainted, costumes can be altered or taken apart completely for the cloth in them. This is no small saving—I once built all the scenery for three full seasons of nonmusicals from the lumber used in the staircase for *Hello, Dolly!*—but it is not quite the same as building a set of flats for an interior set and rearranging them with new coats of paint for the next five years, which is the way many community theatres handle their scenic needs for nonmusicals.

A second drawback to rentals is the time during which they are available. If you construct materials yourself, they are available for rehearsal or practice as soon as you finish them. The only way rental costs can be minimized is to minimize the time you use the material. Most groups can't really afford to rent scenery, costumes, or lighting equipment for more than a week before the first performance. This means that there is little time for performers to get adjusted to any odd clothing (such as the Oriental costumes of *The King and I*) or to complex scenery changes.

Third, rentals cannot be controlled. Unless you live in the immediate vicinity of the company from which you rent, all ordering must be done by mail or by telephone. No matter how carefully you order and no matter how carefully the company ships, you still have no idea what the show will really look like until you open the boxes, and at that point it is too late to correct any mistakes or problems. Most of the time, of course, there are no mistakes. But there are always problems.

When scenery is rented from one place, costumes from another, props from a third, and all orders are done from catalog descriptions, there is no guarantee that the pieces will all fit together into a unified show. Costumes in particular are unpredictable. Since you must order by size, there is no likelihood that everything needed will be available in the exact sizes you need. It is not at all unusual to find that for your "Ascot Gavotte" in *My Fair Lady* you have seven gray dresses and one red one because the company ran out of gray dresses in the sizes you need. Nor is it unusual to find chorus costumes that are more flamboyant than the principals' costumes, because the chorus costumes are often randomly selected from any clothes of the period that happen to be the proper sizes. At other times the costumes will look fine but will not quite fit anyone. This is especially common in high school productions because a boy's proportions are different from a man's, so that a size 36 coat may "fit" but still not look right.

Fourth, rental materials are designed for use in "typical" productions of most popular shows. Each rental house will have its own idea of typical, so that some specialize in sets or costumes for enormous stages that try to duplicate the New York production, while others aim for more generalized and simplified materials for organizations with smaller budgets. Drops, for example, come in several standard sizes for typical or average-sized proscenium stages. Unfortunately there are very few such typical stages, and the drops are often too wide, too narrow, too tall, or too short for the stage you will be working on. Costumes are constructed for a variety of uses: Costume houses make an enormous part of their annual income at Halloween, and their stage costumes often reflect this multipurpose usage; costumes for *Camelot*, for example, may be generalized so that they can also be rented out to productions of *Once Upon a Mattress*, any children's fairy-tale productions in medieval settings, and anyone who wants to dress up as a princess or a knight at Halloween.

Fifth, rentals do not eliminate the need for your own personnel. People tend to assume that if they rent sets, costumes, props, and so on, they can eliminate the need for designers and stage crews, thus simplifying the organizational problems for a show. But there still must be someone who decides what to order, makes all the necessary measurements and plans, takes the time to discuss options and make decisions with the rental houses, and knows how to use the rented materials properly to avoid extra fees for damage.

Finally, there is the problem of cost. You can almost always rent sets or costumes for musicals for less than it would cost you to build the same thing. However, if you have enough volunteers and equipment to construct things yourself, you can almost always build something different, but designed especially for your own requirements, for less. Thus, if you want or need your own special look for a show, rentals are not necessarily cheaper.

Rentals will not solve all your technical problems. The decision to rent or not to rent depends on your situation. For some groups renting will be impractical because the stage is too small or ill equipped or the budget is too limited. For others, construction will be even more impractical due to lack of storage space; it is pointless to build scenery and costumes to be saved for future use if you have no place to store them.

In general, the following advice will be practical:

1. If you do only musicals but do them regularly, construct those things that might be reused (drops, basic wagons, standard flats, and so forth) and rent everything else.
2. If you have no storage space, rent. The cost of storage space has to be considered as part of the cost of the scenery and costumes, which often makes local construction more expensive than rental would be.
3. If you are a school group with a mixed program of musicals and non-musicals and a commitment to some semblance of education, build as much as possible.
4. If you want complete artistic control of the production, build everything.

A reminder: If you rent, you must know *exactly* what you need. This means you must prepare in the same detail as if you were designing and constructing materials for yourself. The rental house will not know what to send unless you tell them what you need and what size you need it in. In particular be aware of the details of costumes. Don't just order suits, for example, because that's what you'll get. If you need ties, collars, cuffs, false shirt fronts, suspenders, or cuff links to go with those suits, be sure to order them too or you could get a big surprise when you open the boxes.

Fee reductions

Some groups try to reduce their royalty or rental fees by asking for reduced royalties because they are nonprofit or charitable organizations. Most of the time this is a pointless argument. All amateurs are nonprofit or charitable organizations of some kind. As high as royalties may seem, they are normally quoted with that assumption in mind. In some rare cases, such as performances for charity patients who cannot pay admission or at a play festival from which you receive no income, some agencies may reduce or eliminate royalties, so it may be worth your effort to try. In general, however, the attitude of the agency is that every performance in some way reduces the value of the work; even if you charge nothing, the people who see your show will be less likely to pay to see someone else's production somewhere else. Hence, the agencies and the people they represent tend to expect to be paid for their material whether or not you expect to be paid for it.

Some groups try to reduce rental fees by copying parts. Photocopying parts is always illegal. If you need more copies, buy or rent them.

Some groups try to reduce their fees by lying or stealing material. In general, this takes two common forms. The group may request material for three performances and then give six, thereby paying half the normal royalty. Or in some cases they simply steal everything by copying the script from a library and staging the show without paying any royalties at all. This is an abominable practice in all ways. The agencies try to protect their properties in a number of ways, from the use of sides to confuse copyists to the use of clipping agencies that pick up newspaper stories all over the country checking for unauthorized performances. I have met people who have stolen material like this over the years; in almost all cases they were eventually caught, which meant they had to pay both the unpaid royalty and significant additional fines for copyright violations. And when they did get caught, the organizations for whom they had tried to save the money claimed they knew nothing about it and left the individual to pay the fines out of his or her own pocket. With the current increased pressure on all copyrights caused by photocopying machines and video-cassettes, copyright holders are much more sensitive to this problem than they were even a decade ago and much more likely to prosecute to make an example. Even if the morality of such theft doesn't bother you, don't do it. Save your money in other ways or find another show.

ACCOUNTING

No matter how meticulously the budget is prepared or how accurate its estimates, it has no meaning without sensible and simple accounting procedures. There must be a way for someone to know at any moment how much has been spent, how much is still available, and how much must be saved for future expenses. This not only keeps things organized but is also the only way to be ready for the inevitable emergencies that will arise in the course of any production.

Purchase Orders

Most groups build their budget control around the purchase order (PO). This is a basic form by which material is ordered from a business with a promise to pay upon presentation of a bill from that business. Any person with a purchase order in hand may actually make the purchase; then the business sends a copy of the PO and a bill to the financial officer of the organization. Because the PO indicates the maximum price to be paid, the business manager knows how much money has been committed to each purchase before the purchase is actually made and is thus able to keep within the budget.

The PO system, however, is a bulky and awkward one with several important drawbacks for a theatrical group. First, it requires an enormous amount of time: The purchaser shops and finds the material and the company with the best price, then requests a purchase order, after which the business manager issues a PO. Then the purchaser goes back to the business and gets the supplies, after which the business sends the PO to its own accounting department, where a bill is issued and mailed, following which the original organization sends the bill through channels until a check is issued and returned to the company involved. The cumbersome nature of this process adds enormously to its expense. The purchaser invariably misses all sales or other bargain situations because there are so many steps involved. The process is so complex that issuing the PO itself costs money (from $5 to $10 each depending on the organization) in various administrative expenses for both the issuing organization and the business firm involved. This in turn means that many smaller businesses will not accept purchase orders. Sadly, although the PO should enable you to predict the exact cost of items, many businesses have learned that, due to the time between shipment and payment, bills can be inflated above the estimate. Since the ordered items have been used by then, they cannot be returned and the inflated bill must be paid.

Charge Accounts

Some organizations try to eliminate the complexity of the PO system by establishing charge accounts with specific businesses. Unfortunately, this eliminates the business manager's ability to oversee expenses. The budget can be completely destroyed before any bills arrive, and nothing can be done about it. It also limits the organization to a few businesses where they may or may not actually find what they need at the best price. In addition, the number of local businesses that are not part of larger chains has declined dramatically in recent years, so that there are few such businesses that allow such regular charge accounts.

Petty Cash

Either purchase orders or charge accounts will work for rental orders and bulk items such as lumber or costume material. But many of the things you will need are one of a kind and can be purchased from only one place or in small and inexpensive units. Many other items are needed immediately—if you run out of nails on Saturday while the stage crew is working, you don't have the time to fill out a PO, turn it in on Monday, wait a week or so to get it back, and then go get the nails; you need them right now. For these kinds of purchases you need a functioning petty cash fund. This has to be a much larger fund in a theatrical production than in most other situations. Hundreds of dollars will circulate through petty cash simply because that is the only way many purchases can be made. Thus it is not a miscellaneous category for paper clips and coffee, as in an office, but rather a convenient way to make significant purchases.

Most organizations maintain control over petty cash by reimbursing individuals rather than issuing the cash in advance. When the shop runs out of nails, the TD goes down to the hardware store and buys some, then turns the receipt in and is reimbursed. There are usually limits on how much can be reimbursed at any one time. This encourages people to turn their receipts in immediately so that the records can be kept up to date and prevents one person from committing the organization to a large, unexpected expense. I have run complete productions on petty-cash systems and find that they work well. At first glance this system seems to be open to manipulation and fraud, but in my experience I found far less than occurred with PO-billing systems.

Budget Control

Whatever system or combination of systems you use, the business manager should be at every production meeting (or brief the producer before each meeting) to report on the exact state of finances at that time. The business manager should never be able to veto a production expenditure, but he or she should be able to hold any questionable expenditures until specifically discussed and approved during a production meeting.

The production staff may change the budget by shuffling funds around and modifying the production in some way. However, it is essential that the state of the entire budget be considered when any changes are proposed. The business manager cannot simply wait until all the money is gone and then say, "Sorry, no paint for the scenery and no programs, 'cause we're out of money." The first expense is not always the most necessary expense; watch the budget at all times, not just when you get near the bottom of the barrel.

5

Planning the Production

While you develop the final budget, you must also organize your production staff and begin detailed preparations and plans for the actual staging of the show. These plans cannot be completed until the budget is done because the final shape of designs will be limited by the amount of money available for them. The nature of the plans will affect the demands made on the budget at the same time. Hence, this planning process will overlap the budgeting process discussed in Chapter 4. For purposes of explanation, however, we will assume that the budget has been established at this point.

PRODUCTION STAFF

In order to get the musical on the stage, you need a production staff, the people who do the planning, preparation, organization, rehearsal, and operation of the individual production but do not perform in it. For people unfamiliar with musical production, the size of this staff comes as something of a shock. A basic list of this staff is shown in Table 1.

Most of these staff members must be found in the local community. Community groups can look to three basic sources: (1) teachers in local schools, especially music and dance teachers, (2) people who have worked on other productions of any kind, especially stage managers and backstage crews, and (3) friends of people already committed to this particular production who dare not refuse to participate. Volunteers round out the positions but usually do not appear until after the show has been cast.

In schools, certain staff positions tend to be treated as givens: The speech or drama teacher serves as stage director; the choir director serves as music director, teaching the songs; the band or orchestra director as conductor; and the dance class teacher from the physical education program as choreographer. This is often not a voluntary arrangement. Almost all other positions can be and usually are filled by students. This places an additional burden on all the adults involved: Students demand more supervision and instruction than would ideal adult staff members, but then such supervision and instruction is part of the educational process of the musical production. With good supervision students can do most of the staff work listed in Table 1. Rarely have I been disappointed by the work of student crew heads or student designers and choreographers—even at the high school level—when they have been properly supervised and guided by the teaching staff. They will not always be brilliant, of course, but even trained and experienced adults do not always do superior work.

In an ideal situation each of these staff positions should be filled by a different person; however, few groups are in ideal situations, and one person may be forced to fulfill several functions.

In schools, typically most duties fall to the stage director, who is usually the drama or speech teacher and who often must serve as stage director, producer, one of the designers, and technical director. This teacher usually performs most of the duties of the business manager as well, with checks and purchase orders issued by the school administrative offices but all budget control left to the teacher's responsibility.

In other situations, the time schedule may allow one person to fill several jobs. For example, the scenery designer prepares designs before the sets are built and thus often has time to act as either technical director or master carpenter or both, supervising the construction and painting of those designs. In similar fashion, the people on

Table 1. Basic Production Staff for Musical

TITLE	DUTIES	SPECIAL SKILLS AND KNOWLEDGE
Producer	☐ Coordinate all staff. ☐ Supervise budget. ☐ Supervise technical organizations ☐ Coordinate and plan production schedule. ☐ Mediate crises.	☐ Organization ☐ Responsibility ☐ Practicality ☐ Sensitivity ☐ General artistic experience ☐ Negotiation skill
Stage Director (Director)	☐ Hold all nonsinging and nondancing rehearsals. ☐ Coordinate singing and dancing rehearsals. ☐ Hold all combined rehearsals. ☐ Define the basic look of show. ☐ Collaborate with other directors. ☐ Develop/encourage acting performances. ☐ Fit all the pieces of the show together.	☐ Experience in theatre ☐ Organization ☐ Imagination ☐ Sensitivity ☐ Ability to work with actors ☐ Ability to communicate clearly with staff
Music Director	☐ Supervise all musical aspects of production. ☐ Plan and organize all musical rehearsals. ☐ Arrange for accompanist. ☐ Arrange for orchestra.	☐ Knowledge of music ☐ General knowledge of musical theatre ☐ Organization
Conductor	☐ Conduct the orchestra in rehearsals and performance.	☐ Read music ☐ Conducting skills
Chorus Master (usually Music Director will also be either Chorus Master or Conductor, or both)	☐ Teach songs to singers.	☐ Musical skills ☐ Ability to work with singers ☐ Ability to teach music ☐ Familiarity with show singing styles
Dance Director (Choreographer)	☐ Design dances. ☐ Teach dances. ☐ Rehearse dancers. ☐ Supervise all "movement" (if agreed).	☐ Knowledge of dance ☐ Ability to teach ☐ Patience ☐ Ability to visualize dance in groups, not solos
Scenery Designer	☐ Plan all scenic elements. ☐ Provide drawings for all scenery to be constructed. ☐ Supervise construction and/or painting of scenery (in most groups). ☐ Arrange rentals where used. ☐ Shop for scenery materials.	☐ General artistic imagination ☐ Knowledge of stage scenic practice ☐ Organization ☐ Dependability ☐ Graphic drawing
Costume Designer	☐ Plan all costume elements. ☐ Provide sketches, patterns, or directions as needed for costume construction. ☐ Shop for costume items and material. ☐ Oversee costume construction. ☐ Arrange rentals where used.	☐ General artistic imagination ☐ Knowledge of costume and clothing techniques ☐ Organization ☐ Dependability

TITLE	DUTIES	SPECIAL SKILLS AND KNOWLEDGE
Lighting Designer	☐ Plan all lighting elements. ☐ Arrange for all lighting equipment. ☐ Plan light cues. ☐ Rehearse light crews.	☐ Knowledge of field ☐ Organization ☐ Taste ☐ Ability to coordinate with others
Sound Designer	☐ Prepare all sound effects. ☐ Plan microphones and sound reinforcement system for production. ☐ Arrange for all necessary equipment.	☐ Knowledge of field ☐ Ability to coordinate with others ☐ Organization ☐ Dependability
Prop Master/Mistress	☐ Procure all props. ☐ Design props not designed by scenery designer. ☐ Find and arrange for borrowed or rental prop items. ☐ Organize and supervise prop crew.	☐ Taste ☐ Knowledge of community resources ☐ Organization ☐ Ability to work with others ☐ Responsibility
Stage Manager	☐ Maintain schedules. ☐ Keep track of the performers. ☐ Prepare prompt book. ☐ Coordinate backstage crews, equipment, scenery, and so forth. ☐ Attend all rehearsals. ☐ Schedule running crews as needed. ☐ Organize all backstage elements. ☐ Call cues for show in performance. ☐ Establish all operating procedures for performances. ☐ Supervise all aspects of actual performance. ☐ Coordinate information from all directors and producer. ☐ Inform cast of all necessary information.	☐ Organization ☐ Responsibility ☐ Imagination ☐ Even temper ☐ Legible handwriting ☐ Ability to read music score ☐ Ability to get along with people
Technical Director	☐ Supervise all technical aspects of stage. ☐ Coordinate all technical aspects of production. ☐ Organize, schedule, and supervise all construction and installation of equipment, scenery, and so forth. ☐ Organize light, sound, and scenery shifting crews (usually).	☐ Detailed knowledge of stagecraft and electronics ☐ Detailed knowledge of facility ☐ Responsibility (On rented stages, a TD often comes with the building; other groups will appoint a production TD just for the show itself.)
Rehearsal Accompanist	☐ Accompany all singing rehearsals. ☐ Accompany all full rehearsals prior to orchestral arrival. ☐ Accompany or provide rehearsal tapes for dance rehearsals.	☐ Piano skill ☐ Reliability ☐ Patience

TITLE	DUTIES	SPECIAL SKILLS AND KNOWLEDGE
Business Manager	☐ Keep all financial records. ☐ Sign checks. ☐ Issue purchase orders (if used). ☐ Set up box-office procedures. ☐ Supervise ticket sales. ☐ Record and deposit all funds earned. ☐ Report on financial status to producer and/or board regularly.	☐ Bookkeeping skills ☐ Honesty ☐ Reliability ☐ Organization
Publicity Director	☐ Plan all publicity for show. ☐ Arrange advertising. ☐ Arrange photos, stories, interviews, and the like. ☐ Arrange for posters, programs, and so forth.	☐ Familiarity with local media ☐ Reliability ☐ Ability to project positive image ☐ Familiarity with graphic arts
House Manager	☐ Arrange for ushers. ☐ Supervise ushers and house staff during run of show. ☐ Open and close house during run. ☐ Supervise intermission sales (if used).	☐ Reliability ☐ Organization ☐ Familiarity with resources of community and organization
Box Office Manager	☐ Organize box-office operations. ☐ Arrange box-office staff as needed.	☐ Reliability ☐ Honesty ☐ Ability to deal with public
Assistant Director	☐ Take notes for director. ☐ Rehearse small groups as needed.	
Assistant Dance Director (Dance Captain)	☐ Drill dancers in routines.	☐ Dance training ☐ Patience ☐ Ability to teach
Assistant Stage Manager	☐ Assist Stage Manager as needed.	☐ Reliability
Wardrobe Master/ Mistress	☐ Supervise all finished costumes. ☐ Unpack, store, and return rental items. ☐ Organize costume areas backstage. ☐ Organize costume changes. ☐ Arrange for cleaning and emergency repairs of costumes.	☐ Organization ☐ Basic sewing skills ☐ Ability to deal with others
Master Carpenter	☐ Supervise all scenery construction. ☐ Supervise all packing and unpacking of rental items.	☐ Carpentry skills ☐ Familiarity with stage practices ☐ Organization ☐ Instructional skill

TITLE	DUTIES	SPECIAL SKILLS AND KNOWLEDGE
Stage Crew Head (often the Master Carpenter or Stage Manager)	☐ Organize scene changes.	☐ Organization ☐ Reliability
Board Operators	☐ Operate light and sound boards during run of show.	
Makeup Director	☐ Organize makeup of cast. ☐ Supervise wigs. ☐ Instruct cast in makeup techniques (where necessary).	☐ Knowledge of makeup techniques
Construction Crews	☐ Build scenery, costumes, props as needed.	☐ Craft skills
Running Crews	☐ Operate backstage during shows as needed (stage crew moves scenery, prop crew moves props, and so forth).	
Ushers	☐ Take tickets at door of auditorium. ☐ Provide programs for audience. ☐ Help audience find seats. ☐ Help maintain organization of house areas during show.	☐ Pleasant appearance
Ticket Sellers	☐ Sell tickets. ☐ Staff box office as needed.	☐ Honesty ☐ Meticulousness ☐ Pleasant appearance

the construction crews who build the sets and costumes before the show opens may also work on the running crews, who move scenery and props and help with costume changes during the run of the show. Although this seems a practical arrangement when a group is short-handed, it is not always successful. Designers, for example, are not necessarily trained in shop operation and may make poorly organized technical directors. Successful combining of positions depends on the skills of the individuals involved.

This is why a person volunteering to fill several positions at once should not always be eagerly accepted. When such people have the skills necessary for both positions their work is often more unified and imaginative than would be likely if such jobs were separated. But if they do not have the necessary skills (which are often quite different), the results can be disastrous for everything except the individual's ego. Everyone with experience in amateur productions has a horror story to illustrate this, so we need not go into detail here. In general, it is wise to be wary of anyone who *wants* to do everything. Many people can do a bit of everything and if pressured by circumstances might consent to do so, but when they are eager to do so, especially on a musical, then that's an excellent sign that you have either someone who does not know what he or she is getting into or an egotist who will create unnecessary problems.

THE CONCEPT

In an ideal situation the stage director is responsible for what is often called the *concept* of the production. The concept is a statement of the basic approach to be used in dealing with the material, a definition of the "look" or the "feel" of the production, or of the particular aspects of the script that the production should emphasize or de-emphasize. A good director, however, develops this approach through discussion and persuasion rather than dictation. Impressions and suggestions from all members of the creative staff are considered and absorbed, along with the director's own study of the script, and then connected, modified, and organized into some idea or visual image that can help keep the production unified.

For the amateur musical producing group there are numerous limits on the development of a concept that are not present for non-musical productions. You are working with established material, rather than new, unknown material. In addition, there are strict contractual limits on what you can or cannot change from the original productions (which we will examine later in this chapter). Finally, the audience expectations are important because the show as played in New York is widely documented in cast albums and photos and touring companies. All of these considerations militate against any vivid, new interpretive concepts of musicals in the manner of so much contemporary directorial and design work with classics or unknown new plays.

In a very practical sense, the New York orchestrator often sets the concept for the production. You cannot logically do a "punk" *West Side Story*, no matter how attractive an update that might seem, because Bernstein's score and its orchestration are so firmly rooted in jazz music of the fifties. In other shows the design is so closely built into the show that the two are inseparable: *A Chorus Line* without a bare stage, dance rehearsal clothes, and mirrors is no longer *A Chorus Line*. This does not mean you must always seek to duplicate the original New York staging; it merely means that the limits on the organization's plans are much tighter with musicals than contemporary directors are used to dealing with in nonmusicals.

PRODUCTION MEETINGS

Members of the production staff do much of their planning alone. The scenery designer develops scenery plans, the music director analyzes and plans the musical features of the show, and so on; yet, each of these individual functions must be coordinated with the work of everyone else, so that the production fits together. This is done by means of regular production meetings.

A production meeting is simply a regular meeting of the various staff members involved in the planning and rehearsal of the production. Staff members meet, discuss the show, the rehearsal period, problems and solutions, and try to reach practical and unified decisions about the various aspects of the show.

These meetings should begin significantly before the casting of the show and continue on a regular basis—at least once each week—until the opening of the show.

Often such meetings are chaired by the stage director, the person with the ultimate responsibility for the staging of the show. When there is a producer for the show he or she will often preside, but the lines of authority for what goes on the stage still lead back to the stage director.

In general, I have found the following sequence of production meetings to be both practical and valuable.

Stage 1: Analysis

The first full production meeting is a long one, one of the longest you will have, because it is devoted to a detailed analysis of the requirements of the script. All three stage directors, the producer, and any designers involved should be present. If you have a long or particularly complex show, this may take two meetings.

Each person should have read and studied the script prior to the first meeting, looking for those points that apply to each specialty. In other words, the music director should have already analyzed the musical requirements indicated in the score, the scenery designer should have examined the basic practical demands of each setting, and so on.

In the course of this first meeting the staff talks through the entire show, scene by scene. Discuss the practical requirements for each scene, the shape and content, the appearance and changes of the various characters involved, the mood, and potential practical problems that may arise as you try to stage each scene. In all cases at this point, concentrate on analysis of the information in the script. Worry about solutions to problems at a later time; this meeting is to identify the needs and potential problems only. The basic question to ask is, What does the script indicate that the audience should eventually see and understand? How you make all these things clear to the audience cannot be decided in a single meeting.

A basic approach to the production should emerge at the end of this first meeting. If there are disagreements about what should be stressed in the script, about what the audience should see or experience, the director must indicate the basic concept that somehow will unify or resolve these disagreements. This concept may at this point be fairly generalized, but it should indicate the way in which the group expects to go.

Stage 2: Design

In the second stage of production meetings you will develop the practical plans for the production. In general, these should evolve over several different meetings about a week apart.

Essentially, the same people who were at the first meeting should be a part of all these sessions. The business manager should be added to offer financial advice where needed, if there is no producer. If there is a stage manager known at this time, he or she should also attend; the earlier the stage manager knows what the show will ultimately look like, the better he or she will be able to organize the operation of the backstage areas.

When we call this the design stage, we obviously indicate the development of scenery and costume designs; however, this is also the period when the stage director and choreographer begin their staging plans as well, so that their plans can be compared and coordinated to the designs of the other participants.

The first of these meetings generally involves the presentation of rough sketches based on the information and discussion at the last analysis meeting. The scene designer will show and discuss a rough sketch, discuss colors or styles intended, and so on. Others will comment and question as the ideas relate to their parts of the show, their understanding of the concept to be used in the production, and their practical requirements. The costume designer will go through the same process, showing rough sketches of a few major costumes, indicating the approach, style, color palette, materials, and so forth. Again the group will discuss these as they apply to specific problem areas and to the general understanding of the approach to be used in the production.

At this point there are usually still a number of tentative ideas and generalized points to clear up. Most often each person in the group will have left the first meeting with a concept expressed in words, which they then interpret in completely different ways. When the first rough sketches come back, the director can see that each person has a different idea of what something "bright" or "jazzy" in fact is. By using the rough sketches as something concrete to point to, the group can come to a more specific understanding of the concept involved. At the end of this meeting everybody will go off to work individually with a much clearer understanding of the way the show should look and feel.

The second design meeting will again deal with rough sketches, but usually in more quantity. If in the first meeting the designers showed sketches for a few key sets and a few key costumes, at this one they will show sketches for most of the sets and most of the costumes or at least for representative costumes from each of the scenes.

Because the basic concept is clearer at this time, the work can be more detailed and/or extensive. Again the whole group discusses the designs in relation to their special requirements. In particular be especially aware of the financial ramifications of these plans. If the ideas are not likely to fit within the potential budget, then the plans *must* be modified early. By the end of this meeting, some decision should be reached as to whether these are in general what is needed and which specific modifications need to be made.

A note of advice for directors in particular: These are meetings, not examinations. Many directors tend to approach the meetings with the design staff as if they were administering tests that the designers must pass or fail by somehow guessing what the director wants to see. Development of designs is a process of interchange by which the generalized verbal ideas and the specific practical requirements of the script are reinterpreted in concrete visual forms. It takes a great deal of discussion to make sure that the visual form is a valid translation of the verbal form, but there are many valid translations. The designers are not merely desk jockeys who do the practical work for the director's designs; they are specialists and creative people who use a slightly different form of expression and should be treated as such.

Design meetings should continue until the final designs are developed and approved by the director. In the future, however, such presentations will be a part of production meetings that must also be devoted to other questions.

Stage 3: Scheduling

Once the basic approach to designs has been established and accepted, the production staff must establish a production schedule. This is a master calendar for all aspects of a production from the initial planning stages through the final postproduction meetings and clean-up sessions. It should indicate the general shape of rehearsals, although a detailed rehearsal schedule will not be developed until after casting is completed.

The complete production schedule shows the date, place, and time for every intended activity in the process of production. This includes the following:

- Ordering scripts
- Expected receipt of scripts and scores
- Announcement of auditions
- Regular production meetings
- Auditions
- Beginning of rehearsal period and general rehearsal times (that is, evenings, afternoons, weekends, places needed for such rehearsals, and so forth)
- Orchestral meetings and rehearsals
- Deadlines for ordering materials and rentals
- Expected arrival of rentals and materials
- Construction work
- Publicity sessions
- Photo sessions
- Deadlines for technical items and installations
- Move-in to theatre space
- First meetings of various crews
- Ticket sales
- Technical and dress rehearsals
- Performance
- Major social functions (cast parties, fundraising sessions, charity performances, and the like)

This schedule has no value if it is not realistic, so be sure to plan it with careful attention to detail. Before the schedule is finished it should be considered in a production meeting that includes all the known production staff—directors, designers, crew heads, TD, publicity director, and so on.

Be sure to note on the schedule the dates at which actions must be initiated as well as when they must be completed. If a costume supplier says "Allow ten days for shipping and handling," then be sure to mark the order deadline at least ten days before the day you actually want the costumes.

Finally, remember that the schedule has no value if no one knows what it is. Do not make one copy and post it on the office wall and expect everyone in the show to come by the office daily to check on it. Post it in some place where everybody will have an easy opportunity to see it regularly. Even better, make copies of it so that everyone on the staff at least has a personal copy.

Stage 4: Final Agreement

Before rehearsals begin there must be one final meeting at which the precise concept for the show is clearly formulated and accepted. This meeting should include all three directors, the producer, the designers, and the stage manager. At this meeting, finished designs, which have been shown and discussed in various stages in earlier meetings, are presented for approval by the stage director. Then, the entire show is talked through again in light of the plans being made for the actual staging.

Each scene is discussed, one by one, in relation to the designs and to the various directors' plans. The choreographer indicates the kinds of dances planned, the stage director the shape of the show's staging so that the choreographer knows where numbers must begin and end. The music director indicates problems and learns what the singers will probably be asked to do while they are singing. All of these are related to the space available in the finished set design and to the look and feel of the show indicated in all of the various designs.

This is an essential meeting and another long one. Any questions that the three directors may have about any point in the production should be answered (as far as can be answered before the cast starts rehearsals and orders are made or construction work begun). In this way the music director will not be caught off guard later when he comes to a dress rehearsal and finds that all the tenors aren't standing together; the stage director can find out that it is impossible for singers to sing standing on their heads and eliminate such business before wasting time in rehearsal; and the choreographer can see the clothes the dancers will be wearing and the background of scenery against which they will be moving, which will seriously affect the shape and detail of the dances. Without this final coordination and understanding the rehearsals will be a mess. Each director and designer will go off into their own area of specialization for the next few weeks; if this specific coordination is not established now, it most likely will never be established.

Stage 5: Rehearsal Problems

Once rehearsals begin, the full production staff should meet regularly, about once a week, to discuss the various aspects of the rehearsal period. At this meeting each person will report on the progress made in each part of the production since the last meeting and will raise problems for discussion and solution. The stage director will announce or agree to suggested modifications in plans for any relevant areas of the production, the producer or business manager will receive any bills or orders that must be recorded or paid, and a regular update on the state of the budget should be given to all concerned.

These meetings are essential to the development of a good production. Only through such meetings will everyone know how the show is going, and only here can everyone hope to understand the many necessary changes in original plans.

Clout

In every organization some people have more power, authority, and influence than others. Musical productions are no different. There must be people who make decisions. Unfortunately they are not always the people who are supposed to make those decisions. Whatever title such a person might have, nothing happens without at least the tacit approval of the person with the clout. In the professional theatre, clout may lie with any number of different people, depending on the show. In some shows it may lie with the producer, while in other cases the producer may defer to a director. In many cases everyone defers wherever possible to the star, whom they think is essential to the show's success: If the star wants another song, the show is rewritten to take a song from a supporting player and give it to the star; if the star doesn't like his or her costumes, they are changed, and so on.

Amateur productions will often have even more jockeying for position because clout itself is the only significant pay for many in the staff and cast. This becomes especially evident in production meetings where decisions must be made, and a significant level of tension can accompany these meetings if the following points are not clearly understood by all members of the staff.

Role of the producer

The producer for an amateur production serves a far different function than a producer for a professional production. Professional producers have money at risk for potential profit and thus generally exercise the authority that goes with that investment. When particular expertise is needed, they can hire that expertise from a large pool of talent and experience. Although the amateur producer also represents an organization at financial risk, he or she must draw expertise from a much more limited talent pool and rarely if ever can afford to hire such expertise at its real value. The professional can hire a new designer if problems arise, but the amateur who demands that scenery be done a certain way may suddenly find that he or she soon has no scenery. The amateur producer is not the boss but rather the coordinator. It is an important distinction.

The producer does have one significant decision-making role in the successful amateur production of musicals. As the representative of the organization and the person responsible for the budget, he or she should have veto rights over *changes* in production decisions made *after* the budget has been officially established. If the director and set designer decide during the third week of rehearsals that the show needs an extra set involving six neon signs that will cost a thousand dollars each, the producer can and should say no. Professional productions can continue to add expense in the hope that the possible long run of the show will eventually recoup the outlay; amateur productions invariably have fixed runs, so there is no way to add an extra week's run to pay for this extra expense. The producer should not try to tell other staff members what to design or to build but should have veto power over any changes that might destroy the budget for the production.

Role of the director

As the person ultimately responsible for getting the show on stage, the stage director must have the ultimate authority in staging the show. Difficulties arise from two different misinterpretations of that.

On the one hand, some directors expect to be able to demand that everything be done exactly as they dictate. To a certain extent this may be possible in a nonmusical production, especially in schools where the actors are also the director's students. It is all but impossible in a musical production. The stage director establishes the framework within which all the other directors and designers (and performers) must work and may make suggestions about the best way for each specialist to fit within that framework. But the successful musical director cannot tell those other directors how to actually do their jobs. A good director will tell the music director that a song needs to be faster (and why) or explain to the choreographer how the dance number should fit into the scene in which it is placed or provide the basic concepts and practical requirements for the various designers. He or she will not call rehearsals without the music director and tell the singers to do the song faster or demand that the choreographer insert a specific routine or give the designers rough sketches to simply fill in. The staff are all associates, not servants.

On the other hand, many staff members in a musical production come from backgrounds where they have always been The Authority and thus have great difficulty in surrendering any of that authority. This is especially common in schools and church groups. For example, the music director will usually be the choral director who has always made all the necessary decisions about how the music should sound, how the singers should look in performance, and so on. Then when he or she comes to a musical rehearsal and sees that the stage director has told the singers to move around during a song or to wear a different kind of costume than he or she likes or to interpret the song in a different fashion, frustration and confusion may often lead to open conflict.

The stage director must have the authority to get the show together. It will not come together in any plausibly consistent fashion otherwise. A good stage director will learn ways in which to establish that authority without dictating in other people's areas of expertise, but he or she should never relinquish that final authority. At the same time the various other staff members must learn to relinquish some portions of their traditional authority in order to keep the staff functioning. Eventually someone must have the final say, and that person should be the stage director. Only with such agreements and understandings can any group hope to survive the complex musical production process.

CUTS, ADDITIONS, CHANGES

Any production group will face a significant amount of tension when they attempt to balance their understanding of the script, the actual capabilities of the company, the facilities available for performing, and the expectations of the audience. One of the most common ways to lessen such tension is to change the script in some way.

Most contracts will include a clause that says "No changes may be made without the written consent of the authors or their agents" or words to similar effect. But what this means is not at all clear. No musical script can ever be performed exactly as it was done in New York. In fact, from the moment the show opened in New York, it began to change. Different performers, different lighting operators or pit musicians, and different audiences bring about constant modifications. In the light of that experience, what in fact constitutes a change? If the show originally used drops and you have no fly space for drops, does that mean you can't use any other approach to the staging? If you have to use a smaller cast, can you condense or double (have one performer play two roles) a few smaller roles? Can you change a male role to a female role when you don't have a competent male for the role? Can you cut a few four-letter words to avoid community concern or complaints? These are all common problems, and if you can't make such changes, no musical would ever get produced. At the same time you have both a legal and an ethical requirement to produce the show you advertise.

In general, most agencies interpret this clause to mean no "unreasonable" changes. This begs the issue in many ways because we still have to define unreasonable. Although I cannot claim to offer legal advice that would apply in all cases, most amateur groups are able to make changes and modifications as long as they do not destroy the essential fabric of the show.

Most commonly, most amateur groups shorten all dance numbers and production numbers—with one exception. If the dance carries part of the story line, it cannot be shortened without serious damage to the plot or the shape of the show as a whole. For example, the dream dances in *Oklahoma!* are essential to the emotional tensions among the characters and must be performed as indicated. Production numbers, however, can almost always be shortened with not only little damage but often with actual improvement. As discussed earlier, the key to most production numbers is their sense of excess, and for groups with limited dancers or finances or both, it is often better to stop when you've gone as far as you can go. However, no matter how pointless any number may seem, it may not be cut; if there seems to be no point, it is because you haven't yet found it, not because it isn't there.

If in fact you decide to cut part of a production number, always cut a section in the middle of the number. Remember that the point of the number is its gradual growth to a big finish, so make sure you use the biggest musical finish possible in the number to match the biggest finish you can stage. Never eliminate only the last half of a number when your dancers or choreographer have run out of steam, because that's exactly what the number will look like to the audience.

School groups usually feel they must cut all four-letter words and any particularly suggestive sexual material. Here again the accepted practice is to allow the cutting of a word or even occasional line, but only if it does not signficantly affect the shape of the show. Some lines carry more weight than others—at the end of *My Fair Lady*, Higgins says/sings: "Damn, damn, damn, I've grown accustomed to her face." To have him say, "Darn, darn, darn . . . " would be ludicrous for his character in that situation; if you can't allow Higgins to say "damn," you shouldn't be doing *My Fair Lady*. Within the past few years a number of schools have faced considerable community opposition from productions of *Pippin* and have tried to produce "clean" versions of the show. But it would seem to most reasonable persons that a *Pippin* without its vulgarity is hardly *Pippin* any longer, any more than you can still claim to be doing *The Fantasticks* without the rape song ("It Depends on What You Pay"), *Funny Girl* without "You Are Woman, I Am Man," *Guys and Dolls* without the striptease in "Take Back Your Mink" and Adelaide's role as Nathan's mistress, or *Grease* without the assault on Sandy's virginity. If you expect to cut these kinds of elements in such shows, you must seek approval from the agents, and in most cases you can expect not to get such approval. If you have to cut such essential elements, then you should not be doing the shows to begin with.

Staging may almost always be adjusted to fit the requirements of a particular theatre building; however, no new staging concepts are allowable without approval. You may not shift *South Pacific* to the

Vietnam war, shift *Carousel* to a modern southern carnival, or costume *Camelot* in the manner of the Kennedy family without significantly changing the material. No matter how valid such concepts may seem to you, they are so significant as to require the approval of the copyright holders. You may think your production has little impact, but every production in some way affects the reputation and the potential value of the material, and the people who own the property want to see that value protected. They may love your idea and agree or may hate it and refuse permission, in which case you must surrender either the concept or the show.

One other area often brings the amateur into the realm of the illegal: the interpolation of songs not originally in the show. Unless you have full approval of all interested parties for such interpolations, you leave yourself open to significant legal problems. When you sign a contract for a show, you sign and pay for the dramatic rights to only those songs in the show; any other songs still have "dramatic" rights that belong to the individual copyright holder, who is often a different person or company for each and every song. To interpolate a song you must have the permission of both the owner of the show that will be changed and the owner of the individual song that will be added (and which, if agreed to, will also require an additional royalty payment). This is especially tempting when a show has gone through a significantly different movie version such as *Cabaret, Funny Girl*, or *Grease*. In many cases people want to add the songs that were added to the movie because they are good songs as well as widely known. Such interpolation without permission is illegal in every possible way; the only possible advice is, *don't do it*.

Whenever any cuts or alterations are planned, they should be made during the planning stages and carefully discussed in production meetings. The cut that simplifies life for the dancers may complicate life no end for the costume designer who suddenly does not have enough time for the principals to change costumes during the song, or for the stage manager who needs time to set up backstage for the next scene change, and so on. In this way, everyone begins rehearsals with exactly the same script, and no one wastes valuable time working on material that has already been cut from the show.

ORCHESTRATION

One of the most significant decisions to be made in planning is the choice of orchestration. This is both an artistic and a budgetary decision.

There is probably no more exciting moment in the theatre than that moment when the house lights dim and the orchestra starts the overture. Most people feel a tingle of excitement and eager anticipation, but this only happens if the orchestra can in fact play the music. A weak orchestra can hurt a show in a number of ways. First, it will make it hard for the singers to sing securely because they can't always be sure the orchestra is playing the right notes or will respond at the right tempo or volume. Second, it will make the show seem bad even when it is good. Audiences are very unforgiving to orchestras; where they will forgive and even encourage a singer who misses a note or an actor who drops a line, they will be upset and disturbed by an orchestra that plays out of tune or with no feeling. They take the orchestra for granted and usually only notice it at all if it is bad. Thus you have no choice in this area—if you intend to have a full pit orchestra, it *must* be good.

This problem is increased by the peculiar nature of the pit orchestra itself. To reduce costs in New York, the pit orchestra is always reduced to its absolute minimum size. As a result, four to eight string players are expected to balance against full brass sections. This feat requires superb, solo quality string players. In addition most wind, reed, brass, and percussion players will be expected to play several different instruments; a clarinet player in one number may have to play saxophone in another, then oboe for eight bars in a third. And all the players are terribly exposed—because all are soloists on their instruments, every mistake is heard immediately.

As a result, amateur groups find themselves with real problems. Schools may have orchestras, but those orchestras are usually composed of inexperienced student players who are technically not yet up to the demands of the music; yet the school is under an obligation, both educational and social, to use the orchestra in the musical. Other schools have only bands, so no string players are available at all. Theatre groups in small communities may have no musicians in town at all or no budget to hire competent professionals. Thus music directors inevitably look for ways to simplify the orchestra.

Most shows come with a basic orchestration, so you can see exactly how many players you need when you examine your perusal script and score. You can expand the orchestration, of course, simply by renting extra parts if you have room in your orchestra pit. Many schools in particular will do so by adding separate players for clarinet and saxophone rather than asking a single player to play both, and so on. It is very difficult to reduce the basic orchestration because this was the minimum possible when the show was originally staged. If you eliminate the strings, for example, and try to depend only on the wind and brass players, you may find whole sections of songs unaccompanied; even more important, you will change the musical texture of the show, making it into something different from what it can and should be.

There are several alternatives, if your budget allows. For schools the best approach is to use as many student musicians as possible and then augment them with a few key professionals, especially in the string section. For community groups in a large house, find the money; do not assume that you will find volunteers for this, because you usually won't. Orchestra players know that they will get no credit or acclaim, probably will not be noticed except when they make a mistake, and will have to work very hard. If they have done it voluntarily in the past, they will almost never do it again without payment.

If neither of these methods is practical, the alternate choice (which most licensing agencies encourage) is to use piano accompaniment, or a piano combo that consists of piano and percussion. This is practical because the show is usually rehearsed with piano and it keeps the orchestra at a size that fits even the smallest rooms and budgets. On the negative side this always seems a bit tacky to audiences except in very small theatres; the thrill of the orchestra just isn't there. In recent years this alternative has opened up with the availability of a number of electronic keyboard instruments that can approximate sounds of other instruments quite effectively. Thus it is conceivable that with the right equipment and two or three keyboard players and some percussionists, you can produce a full sound approximating that of an orchestra. Such combo arrangements are most effective in small theatres. When you get into large auditoriums of a thousand seats or more, small combos still feel wrong for most shows.

Whatever you decide, decide it early. Do not begin rehearsals without a commitment from the required orchestral players. This way, if you can't put together a full orchestra, you will know far enough in advance to plan an alternate orchestral sound. Don't assume you will find the players you need and not worry about it until a week before the show opens; that way, you will almost always end up with no orchestral players.

AUDIENCE EXPECTATIONS

One of the most persistent problems facing the production staff when planning a production comes from the familiarity of most musicals. Because the material is both well-known and extremely popular, the audience has very detailed expectations about what they can and should see on stage. These expectations may severely limit what the various directors can or may want to do in this particular production.

Some of these expectations have to do with individual performances. If the audience knows a show was done for or with a particular star, then they will expect to see something related to their image of that star. Your *Funny Girl*, for example, will be expected to act and sing like Barbra Streisand, even though the script keeps claiming the show is about Fanny Brice.

In many cases these expectations concern some physical aspect of the production. Dolly Levi, for example, is expected to wear a spectacularly gaudy red dress because Carol Channing wore such a dress, although that violates every other fact known about her in the script. In some cases the show is based on widely known sources—the costumes for *You're a Good Man, Charlie Brown* or *Li'l Abner* are essentially determined by the comic strips on which they are based; to change them would destroy any sense in the production.

The most destructive expectations, however, are based on the movie versions of the musicals. Most famous musicals have been made into movie musicals, and the movies are always significantly different; yet, for most of the performers and the audience the movie is what they have seen, and thus the movie is what they expect to get when they audition or buy a ticket. Probably the most complete alteration came in the film version of *Cabaret*, in which the major plot elements of the stage play were all but eliminated, transforming the original stars into almost unseen and definitely unsung bit players. The result was a brilliant movie musical, arguably one of the finest ever made. But if you want to do *Cabaret*, you will have to do the stage version, just as you must do for any other show.

Finally, the audience will also often have general expectations about musicals as a whole that can affect their response to your particular show. For example, if the audience comes to the theatre expecting all musicals to have plenty of spectacle, your production of *The Fantasticks* will disappoint them no matter how well done it might be. If they expect musicals to be light, "meaningless" entertainment, a good production of *Company* may leave them highly frustrated.

As can be seen from some of the examples selected above, many audience expectations have little to do with the show that is actually in your script; nevertheless, these expectations are a factor in your planning and must be considered.

Two particular dangers arise, however. First, you may misunderstand the expectations of your particular audience, which is often either more sophisticated or more ignorant than you think. This is especially common in schools, where the bulk of the audience is so young. *The Sound of Music,* for example, was filmed in 1965 and may be fresh in the minds of most teachers and parents, but none of today's high school students were born before 1965 and few are old enough to remember any details even from the movie's many television showings. Thus the expectations you think they have are in fact not present. Second, the production staff must be careful that they do not unconsciously share those same expectations. You are producing the show indicated in the script, not the show you have an idea might be there.

When planning the show, you may accept or ignore these expectations. Most of them, when accepted, will not harm your production except the attempt to reproduce the movie version on stage. At the same time you may logically choose not to meet these expectations. You may just as easily put Dolly in a green dress as a red one. Except for those changes that violate your contract or copyright laws, you are free to reexamine and restage material in many different ways. The recent rock-star version of *Pirates of Penzance* completely violated all the traditional staging practices of that show. Whether the results have anything to do with Gilbert and Sullivan is open to debate, but there can be no doubt that the new approach to the material was successful with audiences.

If you wish to go against these expectations, you must be absolutely authoritative. There can be no halfway measures. Whether you try to duplicate the New York production or completely rethink and restage the entire show, the more you move away from traditions and audience expectations, the more convincing your production must be. It is unfortunate but nonetheless true that if you violate such expectations with the slightest bit of hesitation or suggestion of budget scrimping, the audience will almost always assume that you didn't do it "right" because you didn't know how rather than because you chose to do it in a different way.

6

Casting

Good casting for a musical production can be almost as complex as actually rehearsing the show. The requirements for most musical roles are so demanding that few performers are ever ideal, even at the highest paid professional levels (note the number of musical movies made in which the principals' voices are dubbed by other singers or their dancing done by stunt doubles). Thus it should come as no surprise that most amateur producing groups who have access to only a limited talent pool—those performers in a specific school, church, or local community—may have difficulties in finding an ideal cast for their production. This does not mean that amateur productions must be done poorly or that there is a shortage of talent for them; it simply means that particular care must be taken to match the available performers with the requirements of the musical selected for production.

Most people think casting is essentially simple: You hold auditions and cast the best performers in the principal roles, the next best in the next largest roles, and so on until you reach the worst, who are tucked away somewhere in the chorus. Unfortunately, all too many shows are cast in this way, with the result that many productions make no sense to the audience. Good casting is a detailed and thoughtful procedure, because it matches available roles to the talents and strengths of particular local performers rather than to their ego and status.

WHO CASTS?

It is essential for any good musical production that all three directors together, and only those three persons, decide on the casting.

Many groups tend to split the casting decisions, with the stage director casting the principals, the music director the singing chorus, and the choreographer the dancers. This is especially common in schools where the chorus will tend to come from the students in the choir and the dancers from a dance or movement class. Shows cast in this way usually face unnecessary problems during rehearsals because the people cast have made no commitment to the show; being in the class got them the part, and so they tend to treat rehearsals like classwork. In addition, many cast members will not understand or recognize the authority of other directors: the singers, for example, know only the music director, and thus when they are given directions by the stage director or choreographer, they tend to ignore them. Similarly, the other directors are unfamiliar with the various cast members' talents and may not even know their names, with the result that both plans and rehearsals are awkward. This doesn't even consider the possible conflicts when the choreographer wants a lead dancer whom the music director wants singing a different role, and so on.

Some organizations go to the other extreme and use casting committees. This is always disastrous for three simple reasons. First, the more people involved in a decision, the harder it is to reach a decision all will accept. Second, the people on the casting committee go home after casting and are never seen again, while the directors have to stay and work with the cast. This gives the directors a sense of responsibility and attention that no casting committee could ever provide. Finally, casting is a tremendously social process in even the best amateur groups. So much seems to be at stake for the performers during auditions; so many people want so few glamorous roles that there will be a lot of personal tension and conflict. A casting committee invariably increases that conflict, because people on the committee inevitably talk about the process; soon gossip spreads, cliques form, and jealousy increases. Avoid such committees.

CHOOSING THE CAST

There will be disagreements among the three directors about the best way to cast the show, even at the best of times. But disagreements can be minimized when the auditions are approached in a detailed, organized fashion. If you follow the steps in this section, the three directors can quickly and easily determine the best possible cast for your production.

Step 1:
Analyze the Roles

Before auditions, all three directors should meet and determine the detailed requirements for each role in the show. Examine the script carefully and determine the following points.

Age

In schools this is not a factor, because all ages must be indicated by makeup and costume rather than by performer's age. In other groups where you have casts of mixed ages, it will be extremely important.

Singing range

In practice, this is first a question of sex. Nonmusicals have more leeway in substituting females for males, or vice versa, a common need for groups working from limited talent pools. But in musicals, because most characters sing, roles must be cast to fit within the singing range. This means that male roles stay male, female roles stay female, and crossover roles like Peter Pan will almost always be cast with females rather than small boys because the songs require an adult female singing range.

Determine this range exactly, from the lowest note to the highest in all numbers included in the role. In an emergency you may occasionally change the key of a song to make it lower or higher, but this necessitates recopying all musical parts in the new key, a long and painful process.

Singing style

In most shows a singer will sing only one or two particular kinds of songs such as ballads, patter songs, or "belt" numbers. What type does this person sing and what kind of voice will be needed for such songs?

Personality

What is the basic trait projected by the character? This describes what the character is like most of the time. For example, Jeff in *Brigadoon* makes wisecracks wherever he goes. He does other things as well, but his predominant personality is cynical witticism, although in a friendly, nonvicious manner. This would be the basic personality of the role.

Emotional variety

Are there any points that are significantly different from the dominant personality, something that might require significant acting skill?

Dance

Must the character dance? How much, and in what styles? Must he or she dance and sing at the same time?

Time requirements

In how much of the show does this character participate, and how much rehearsal time is likely to be needed to prepare for it? This is a critical point in amateur groups where people can devote only a few hours a day at best to the production. In *Fiddler on the Roof*, for example, Tevye is in almost every scene and thus will need to be at many more rehearsals than each of his daughters, who are on stage less. However, difficulty of role as well as size must be considered. Normally the most rehearsal time is given to the dancers, who often have no lines at all and may appear in only three numbers; what they do is difficult and takes a long time to learn, and even the quick learners must be present with the group at all times.

Special skills or attitudes

This includes such unusual things as the various circus skills the characters must have for *Carnival!*, for example. It also includes personal mental attitudes. It would be difficult to do *Peter Pan* if Peter is afraid of heights and is terrified of the flying harness. These mental attitudes also include problems that can arise purely because the show is performed in front of friends and relatives. For example, Gypsy in *Gypsy* is a stripper; although she never reaches complete nudity, she does go through the motions and gets close. Whoever you cast must be willing to do this. Some characters must use language that offends some performers, while others express ideas about religion, sex, or society that may upset some people. How far must a performer go to make these scenes effective?

Step 2:
Evaluate Your Analysis

Once the basic requirements of the roles are defined, the three directors must agree on the relative importance of each of these points. This happens in three stages.

Ideal abilities

In general, ideal casting has been considered in Step 1. Your ideal performer can do all the things listed in your analysis of the role. But very often there will be more you wish to add, things that within your concept of the show could be important. For example, is the character physically attractive? Fat or thin? Is there some special skill you would like to add that isn't in the script itself? List all these factors on which the three of you agree.

Minimal abilities

Consider the absolute minimal needs of the role. Can the singing range be modified? If so, in what ways? Can the words of a song be spoken rather than sung? Can the dance number be shortened? Could the character be a different age? Look for what you absolutely must have to be at least acceptable.

Be sure to consider these two points for *all* roles. Chorus members as well as principals have specific requirements. In *The Music Man,* for example, the dancing is done by the kids, so the dancers must look younger than the singers who play their parents. The chorus is supposed to reflect a cross-section of the town, so it should include people of different ages and sexes. These are some of the minimum requirements for these roles.

Prioritized abilities

Which of the ideal requirements is most important? In almost all cases you will not find your ideal. In many cases you will have few auditioners who even meet the minimum requirements. However, there will always be several people for several roles who do meet the minimum requirements but in different ways, so that you can consider some of the ideal characteristics, but a decision can be reached only if you know which of those ideals is most important. For example, in *My Fair Lady* an ideal Higgins would have all the acting skills of a fortyish Rex Harrison while singing somewhat better than Harrison did. However, it is not only possible but necessary to cast the role with someone who does not meet this ideal (remember that even Rex Harrison didn't sing very well). Once you establish what your minimal requirements for the role should be and have people who can meet such minimums, you must determine what is the *most important* factor in this ideal. For my own production, I would rank as most important the ability to speak well and clearly—Higgins makes his living teaching people how to speak, and the plot hinges on that ability; no matter how handsome the actor or how good the singer, nothing will work if he speaks awkwardly or unclearly. This skill supersedes all others, so that I would favor a weaker actor or singer as long as he had this skill. If I had two people of equal speaking skill, then my second priority would be basic personality because so much of the relationship with Eliza depends on his unthinking arrogance. If someone can project that quality in auditions, then I'll find a way to teach them how to sing or act better as we rehearse. Different directors would rank these skills in a different priority, depending on the production. The important factor is not what particular priorities you establish but the fact that priorities have been established before auditions begin.

Be sure that the priorities as well as the ideals and minimum requirements for each role are based solely on your analysis of the script. Far too many organizations miss extremely talented performers because they look only for people who look or sound like the stars associated with a particular role, the singers heard on the cast album, or the performers seen in another production. You are looking for an actor to play Henry Higgins, not Rex Harrison. Be careful not to let the image of Rex Harrison so dominate your thinking that you can't see the auditioners. Cast your production of the show, not someone else's.

Be sure to write these priorities down before you leave this meeting. In the pressure of casting it is easy for one or all of the directors to forget what has been agreed to.

Step 3:
Look for What You Need

Once you have gone to the trouble of defining the requirements of each role and establishing the priorities for the necessary skills, set up auditions to look for what you need. Practical aspects of the audition process itself will be discussed in detail, but it is essential that you remember several points throughout the auditions:

1. You will not find what you need if you don't tell auditioners what you want. Most auditioners will not try to do something in particular unless they think it is expected. You must tell them what you expect to see for each character.

2. You will not find what you need if you don't look for it. Too many directors say they want one thing and then get distracted by a new idea and look for something else in auditions. While the auditions are going on, focus only on what you need.

3. You will not find what you need unless you look at everyone. Many people in amateur productions are too nervous or shy to try for major roles, although they can in fact play them quite well. Your best Higgins may not audition for Higgins, but in his audition for a completely different role or even a chorus part may suggest all the minimum requirements and perhaps even some of the ideals for Higgins. In the same way don't eliminate anyone from consideration while auditions are in progress; when you get ready to cast, you may find that you need that person after all. A community theatre I worked for once hired a director from New York who, used to the large New York acting pool, dismissed people he thought he didn't want as soon as they auditioned. The crisis came when he discovered that he had no one left to play the chorus parts for the show, and only desperate pleading from cast members managed to get back a few of those people who had been so summarily dismissed.

4. You will not find what you want unless all of you watch everything. Even if the choreographer is auditioning dance, the music director and the stage director should observe in order to absorb names, faces, and general impressions of various people and to be familiar with the person when he or she comes up for discussion in the final casting sessions.

Step 4:
Make a Decision

After all the auditions have been seen, the three directors must select the best combination of the available performers for the cast of the show.

In every casting situation the music director naturally wants to cast the best singer, the stage director wants to cast the best physical type and the best actor, while the choreographer wants to cast the most graceful, coordinated person. The only way to focus all these conflicting viewpoints on the show is to establish priorities *before you see the auditions*. By that time you will have already agreed together that some roles must put top priority on certain aspects. Then you can produce a good casting job very quickly and with minimum disagreement.

A certain number of people who audition may not be suitable for any role, but most of the people you are likely to see not only can but also must be cast somewhere. The question is, Where is the best place to put each person so that the best possible show might result?

This question can be broken into two parts: (1) If necessary, who *could* play each role? and (2) Who *should* play each role?

1. Who could *play each role?* Before you make any decisions sit down with your list of minimum requirements for each role made in Step 2. List each role in the show, and beside each character's name list all the people who auditioned and who seem to satisfy these mimimum requirements. Do not evaluate or rank these people in any way; simply list them.

For some roles the list will show a number of competent people. Depending on the show and the size of the organization, you may have as many as a dozen people who could play some of the principal roles and many more who could be in various chorus roles. For other roles there may be only one person who could meet the minimum requirements. Remember, in this stage consider only the minimum, not ideal, requirements for each role.

2. *Who* should *play each role?* First, look at the roles for which no one seems to meet the minimum requirements. Consider your list of priorities made in Step 2. Look through all your auditioners for the person who meets the most of the minimum requirements and your highest ranked priorities. For example, you may have no people the right age for Higgins, but you may have a fine speaker and an okay singer who is only twenty years old. At that point you simply have to take a chance; the age is a low priority in this particular role, so you can cast someone who fits all the other requirements and plan for extra work on the acting and the makeup.

Second, consider all the roles for which only one person meets the minimum requirements. That person is automatically cast, *no matter how good they might also be in a different role*. This is often a traumatic decision, especially since such people will often have a variety of skills. If you are doing *Brigadoon*, for example, Jean *must* dance a serious funeral ballet and a romantic solo number as well; the absolute minimum requirement for the role is that she be a good, trained ballet dancer. In such a case your best-trained dancer must play Jean, although Jean doesn't sing a note, even if she is a fine singer who could play Fiona or Meg terrifically. *You must meet the minimum requirements for each role before you can begin to worry about the ideal.* Always remember that you are casting a complete show, not just a role.

When you have cast the roles for which you had little or no choice, eliminate those people from consideration for all other roles. Usually this will reduce a few more roles to a single choice, and these can now be quickly settled.

Finally, there will be a few roles for which you have several different people remaining who all meet at least the minimum requirements for the part. Of these people, are there any who fit the ideal requirements completely? If so, you are quite lucky, so cast them immediately. In most cases each person will fit some of the ideal characteristics, but not all. At this time turn to your previously agreed-upon priorities and evaluate these people in relation to those priorities. If you have five women who could play Fiona in *Brigadoon* and you all agreed that youthfulness was the top priority for the role, then the one who seems most youthful should be cast. But if you agreed that the quality of the singing voice should be the top priority, then the woman with the best singing voice should be cast, even if the other four women may be younger, prettier, or better actresses.

When you have cast everyone, consider how the cast will fit together. Do romantic couples seem about the same age and size? Do "relatives" resemble each other enough to be acceptable to the audience? Are there enough tenors to balance the altos and sopranos in the chorus? Are there enough members of each sex and/or ethnic group as needed for the script? Will duet voices blend together? And so on. In light of such questions, some modifications of your casting may be necessary.

One important related factor is availability. If you intend to use people with some schedule conflicts, as you often must, you must be sure that they can be scheduled with the other people in their scenes. If your Fiona has night classes on Monday and Thursday, your Jeff has a job where he must work late on Tuesdays, and your Tommy is the director of a church choir that rehearses on Wednesday nights, there will never be a time when they can rehearse together as they must. In such a situation you may have to go to a second or third choice for one or more of these roles.

Alternates

Before you announce the cast, agree among yourselves on an alternate for each role. An alternate need not necessarily be someone who was not cast at all, although it can be. It may be someone in the chorus who could play one of the speaking roles if someone got sick. With luck you will never need to make a cast change, but in most cases you will. In more than eighty productions of my own, musical and non-musical, I have actually opened with the cast I started with fewer than a dozen times, and only once in a musical. People get sick, have family crises, have accidents, even change jobs without warning and leave town. The large casts and long rehearsal periods for musicals increase the chances that such things will happen to someone in your cast. When such problems arise, it helps that all the directors have already agreed as to a probable solution to the casting change; that way, no one panics or is outraged that after spending three weeks teaching a dance or a song, the performer suddenly has to be moved to something else and start over.

There is no need to announce this alternate cast. In a majority of cases no one will be called upon to actually take over a role partway though rehearsal. This is merely another step in coordinating the various directors and guaranteeing that all three of them understand and are working toward the same production of the show.

Understudies and double casting

Because people do get sick, it seems logical to have officially designated understudies who can step in and take over a part. This is essential in the professional theatre, where shows run eight times a week for months at a time. However, it rarely works well in amateur productions.

The directors should have alternates in mind for each role, but it rarely helps to announce these alternates and make them official understudies. First, no matter whom you understudy for, someone else will be the person who gets sick. Second, if the understudy is to be effective, he or she must be rehearsed, which takes extra time and effort for someone who probably will not get to play the part and at the same time takes away from the already limited rehearsal time available to the cast that is designated to perform. Third, it really is not too difficult in most cases to make a cast change during rehearsals if someone does get sick. The old Ruby Keeler plot about the kid who comes out of the chorus to play the star's role when the star breaks her leg is not quite as absurd as it seems. One of the odd things about the rehearsal process is that almost everyone will learn everyone else's part before they learn their own. Someone can come out of one of the small roles and take over a larger role with very little physical rehearsal when you get close to opening night, leaving you with only the small role to teach someone new.

In similar fashion some groups like to double cast some roles, usually the major ones. In this arrangement one set of people plays the leads on Wednesday and Friday, the other set on Thursday and Saturday. This seems like a wonderful idea, but it almost never works. For one thing, double casting means double rehearsals. As a result, instead of one well-rehearsed show, you get two poorly rehearsed ones. Second, it increases company jealousy as members of the two casts constantly compare their performances to each other and drag all their relatives and friends into the competition. The only advantage it has is that it saves the directors from making a hard decision, but directors have to make choices, no matter how hard they might be; that's why there are directors. Make a decision and stick to it, and do the best production you can. That's the reason for holding auditions. It is a tremendous waste of everyone's time and effort if you end those auditions without making a choice.

HOLDING AUDITIONS

The goal of a good audition is to see as much usable material as possible from each potential performer within as brief a time as possible. This requires some careful organization of the auditions themselves.

Preparation

In your announcements of auditions, explain what the show is, how many and what kinds of roles are available, and what you expect people to do at the auditions. In particular specify exactly what you want people to prepare for the audition. If you wish them to sing, indicate the type of song that will be in the style of the show you are doing. For example, if you are doing *Grease* or *Godspell*, tell people to sing a contemporary but melodic number, something with a pop/rock flavor, because that's the kind of music in the shows. If you are doing a traditional Broadway-style show, tell them to sing a standard pop song or a show tune. If doing something more operatic such as *A Little Night Music* or *Little Mary Sunshine*, then they must sing a song that shows off their voices. In general it is best to discourage people from singing a song from the show itself; people tend to precast themselves in a way that limits the effectiveness of their audition when they do so.

Performers must bring their own sheet music for any songs they intend to sing, and the organization is expected to provide an accompanist who can play such music at sight. This is not always easy, and many groups find it more helpful to provide a cassette recorder and ask the auditioners to bring a tape recording of their accompaniment.

In this way the singer is absolutely secure, and the group doesn't have to find the world's greatest pianist. If you choose to do this, however, be absolutely clear that the performer is to provide a tape of the accompaniment, not of a recording with which they will simply sing along.

First Auditions

First auditions are used to narrow the field, not to make final decisions. In general, all you look for is: Who *might* be okay for this production? These auditions usually last several days because there are so many parts to cast and so many people to see. However, they should never take more than three sessions. If you can do it in two sessions, then do so.

There is some valid disagreement as to how the auditions themselves should be conducted. Many people prefer closed auditions, in which the performer is alone with the various directors. In this way there are no distractions and no undue nervousness from a crowd of others watching and listening. However, this really only works if all parts of the audition are done alone, which usually means completely prepared auditions. For most groups such a requirement will scare away almost all the potential auditioners and defeat the purpose of the auditions. Much more practical are open auditions, in which the three directors see auditioners in relatively large groups. This allows you to hear performers read scenes with two or three people at a time, which is both faster and more like what the cast will be asked to do in the show. It also allows you to hold the dance audition in groups, which saves an enormous amount of time for whoever has to teach the initial dance routine. Finally, it gives a chance to see how the performer copes with an audience. In groups of inexperienced performers such as in schools and most community groups, the fact that some auditioners are allowed to see other people audition often seems to encourage the shyer ones to participate as well.

Whatever method is used, every auditioner should do all parts of the auditions, even those who say they can't dance or don't want to sing a solo or act a main role. Many will be too nervous or shy to try for large roles, but few will turn down such a role when it is offered. But you cannot offer a role unless you have seen complete auditions.

General information

Begin each audition by telling all the auditioners what you expect of them for this production: how you see each character, the time requirements of rehearsals, your expectations about attitude and standards, and so on. No one can give you what you want if they don't know what it is. You may do this with a little speech at the beginning, but it is usually better to print it up on a handout given to each person as they arrive.

Singing

Hear each person sing a prepared number. Practically no one can read music any more, which makes it all but impossible to teach a song at the auditions. Thus, if you expect people to sing their best, you must demand that they come to auditions with a song they have already memorized.

Acting

Have each person read a short scene. The acting requirements of most musicals are so eccentric (in the way characters and scenes develop) that traditional audition material, such as monologues from Shakespeare or other playwrights, rarely conveys the brassy, direct, humorous tone of most musicals. Hence, the acting part of the audition must usually depend on some form of cold reading. This is the most awkward part of the audition because the musical script is built around songs, which leaves few short scenes that can be read and still make sense. However, it is not necessary at this stage of the auditions to hear completely developed scenes. There is no reason in first auditions why a scene involving two or three people should ever go more than about two minutes. If there is some potential, it will appear in that time, and usable performers can be called back for more complex material during the second round of auditions.

When scenes are selected for readings, be sure to select them to show what you want to see. If you have decided that in *Brigadoon* you want Jeff's cynical witticism as the first priority, don't audition from the scene after the chase when he isn't cynical or witty.

Dancing

For most amateurs, dancing is even more intimidating than singing; consequently, auditions that demand prepared dance routines will often scare away more potential performers than they bring in. Few people will take the time to prepare dance routines, and even if they do, the routines may have little to do with the style or shape of the production you plan. If you expect to see any dancing, you must be willing to teach a cold routine and then see the people attempt to perform it.

The choreographer or assistant should teach the auditioners a *short*, simple routine, something that you might reasonably expect a coordinated person to learn in ten minutes at most. Then you should see that routine performed. The teaching of the routine can be done in large groups of twenty or so, depending on the routine, but the actual audition performance should usually be done in groups of three to five people. Being in a group gives inexperienced performers some sense of security. At the same time the small group allows you to pay attention to each person and actually see how well they are coping with the demands of the dance.

Time is an especially significant factor in this part of the audition. Some people are slow learners. Professionals are expected to pick up a short routine like this in a very short time, but amateurs will need more. At the same time there is no need to continue teaching until everyone has the routine perfect; they need to know the routine well enough to demonstrate their coordination and grace, or lack of it. But remember, the test of this part of the audition is not the correctness of the routine so much as the impression demonstrated about the dancer by the routine. It is not a routine from the show (it is far too short for that, among other things); it is only a suggestion of the style of routines they might expect to do in the show.

Call-backs

After you have heard all the auditioners, the three directors should confer to consider which people you need to see in more detail. These people are then called back for a second round of auditions on another evening or afternoon.

Call-back auditions serve several important functions and may be used in a number of ways, depending on which of those functions you need at a given set of auditions.

They allow you to see potential performers in more depth. You may ask them to read longer scenes or to prepare scenes from the script so that readings are more nearly like a performance. You may teach them a different and longer dance routine, the better to judge their dance capability.

In some cases, such as very large auditions, this call-back is necessary just to be sure you have the right names attached to the right faces.

Call-backs may be used to compare people. This is especially helpful if you hold initial auditions over several days. Thus, six women who all suggest that they might be able to play a single role might be asked to sing or read a scene from that particular role, one after the other, so that you can see how they compare directly to each other. Call-backs may also be used to establish relationships among potential cast members. Potential Fionas may be read with potential Tommys to see how they look or react as romantic couples. Potential singers can be mixed and matched to see how voices blend for a chorus, duet, or small group. Dancers can be paired to see how they fit as a group or as partners.

Finally, call-backs may be used for something quite minimal and specific. The first round of auditions is an elimination round of sorts, but it is not always necessary to call back everyone who was not previously eliminated unless you actually need to see them for some purpose. There have been shows for which I have been able to cast all the principals at the first round auditions and only called back people for chorus and dance roles. In another I called back five women to go through one simple routine that took less than ten minutes; the role in question needed a particular kind of girlish grace, which initial auditions had not made clear, so we asked each woman to walk, stop, turn, run, stop, twirl, walk, and then sit down, and this constituted the entire call-back. The call-backs are simply an opportunity to see something more or something else from some of the people who auditioned. Their content will vary from show to show.

There is no single best way to plan or organize call-backs, because they serve many different functions. For most normal amateur productions, a first round of auditions taking two or three sessions should be able to handle call-backs in only one more two- to three-hour session. No call-backs should take more than two evenings; that's a clear sign that the directors don't really know what they are looking for.

After the call-backs are completed, the three directors must sit down together with their lists and their priorities and finally make the decision, as indicated in Step 4.

Keeping Organized

From the directors' point of view, the most important part of the audition process is matching names to faces and talents. It does you no good to find the perfect cast if you can't name them so they know to come to rehearsals.

Information sheets

Each person at the audition must complete an information sheet of some kind. These may take various forms; a sample is shown in Figure 9. Any good audition sheet must include the following points:

1. *Identification information*: name, age, sex, personal data such as hair color, height, weight, and so forth. This is not personal data as such (although it will help in some roles to know which persons are tall or short, fat or thin); rather it is the means by which the directors remember who is who. Professionals would also provide a photo, but this is usually impractical for almost all amateur groups. I find it helpful to have people describe their clothes, especially when there are large numbers of auditioners, because it helps me visualize them when I consider the auditions later. (If you do this, remind per-

formers at call-backs or second auditions to wear the same clothes again—it helps the directors remember what they look like.)

2. *Contact information*: address, phone number, and so forth.

3. *Experience*: skills, training, background, and previous performances that might apply to this show.

4. *Availability information*: What commitments and schedule conflicts exist that might interfere in any way with the rehearsal schedule explained at the beginning of the audition or in the handout given to all the auditioners when they arrived? This is extremely important, as it affects not only your schedule but also some of your casting decisions. Be sure that all potential cast members understand that barring emergencies, everyone might be called at any time unless dates of conflict are brought to the directors' attention now. This includes those things to which the person is already committed before accepting a role—business trips, church choir or services, anniversaries or family vacation trips, and so on. (This is always a sensitive area. In an ideal sense, taking a role in the show requires that you give your time to the show. But in a practical sense, performers have personal lives that must be attended to. The most effective approach I have found depends on this information sheet. As a director of the show, I cannot expect people to keep their schedules clear forever just in hopes that they *might* get a part in this show. Thus, when I cast someone, I agree to honor commitments made prior to the time they are cast. In return they agree that the rehearsals now become a prior commitment for anything that arises while the rehearsals are going on.)

5. *Other interests*: Many people who come to auditions just want to be involved in the show. If they don't get a part in the show, they might be willing to work backstage, but they won't commit themselves until they know whether they have a part or not. So always ask somewhere on the form if they have a backstage skill or interest. If they don't get cast, then you can call them up to fill out your production staff and backstage crews; if they get cast, you can put their names in a file to call on for other, later productions.

These information sheets should be handled by one person. Ideally this is the stage manager. However, for many groups the stage manager will not be selected until after the cast is selected because many people will not volunteer to stage manage if they can get a part in the show. Whoever this person may be, his or her job is to see that every auditioner fills out the information sheet and then sort through the sheets

```
                  AUDITION INFORMATION


Name _____ Sex ___

Ht._____ Wt. _____ Hair ____ Age ___ Phone _____

Address _____ Day Phone _____

Parents' Name(s) (for students) _____

Singing Voice: Sop ___ Alto ___ Ten ___ Bar ___ Bass ___
     Singing experience (# of years) School Choir? ___
     Advanced Choir? ___ Church choir? ___ Lessons? ___
     Solos? ___ Other? _____

Dance experience (# of years) Ballet ___ Tap ___ Jazz ___
     Modern ___ Drill team ___ Ballroom ___ Other _____

Acting experience: List recent roles and groups roles
     performed with:




Any other public performance experience:


Rehearsals will be held Mon-Fri, from 7-10pm, ending in
performances for ___ weekends beginning _____ and ending
_____. Please list any commitments or conflicts that you
know of (jobs, family anniversaries, classes, etc.) that
would cause you to miss rehearsals at any of those times:




If not cast, I would like to work on (check as many as you
     like): Stage manager ___ Props ___ Costumes ___
     Scenery ___ Lighting ___ Sound ___ Publicity ___
     House manager ___ Ushering ___ Other _____


Additional information you think we should know about you:
```

FIGURE 9. Sample Audition Information Form

so that the three directors have the correct sheets in front of them during the audition. The directors may make notes on the sheets or in their own notebooks, whichever seems most convenient. But it is essential that they all immediately be able to refer to the audition information about a performer at any time during that person's audition.

Humane auditions

A simple (and thus often overlooked) way to remember who is who is always to call every auditioner by name. When people go on stage for an audition, don't let them begin until you are absolutely sure what their name is. If you have a question for them, always precede the question with their name, and if you give a direction, always include the name in the direction. Some groups develop a theory that making auditioners wear numbers is more professional or somehow more fair, but I have always found it demeaning to the performers and confusing to the directors. There is no place in amateur theatre for the gigantic cattle-call approach to auditions.

Remember at all times that auditions are a cruel process no matter how you hold them. People must put their egos in very delicate and exposed positions. There is simply no reason why auditioners should be belittled or ridiculed for making the attempt, even if they do not make a particularly good attempt. I have seen directors interrupt auditions and tell people to get off the stage, have heard them tell people they have no talent, and have heard them make audible jokes among themselves about the people on stage. This is inexcusable.

Do not string out auditions unnecessarily. Auditoners' nerves can only be stretched so far. Post results as soon as a decision is made or immediately phone people who have been cast. It never hurts to contact the people who were not cast, to thank them for auditioning, to encourage them to try again at the next production, or even to talk them into working backstage. Trying to increase the suspense while postponing an announcement of a decision that has already been made is childish.

The question often arises as to whether you should allow people a second chance. Auditions are complex, and there are often large numbers of people to be seen in a short amount of time. The pressures are enormous. Thus it often seems sensible to have a policy that people can go through the process only once, or that people may audition for only one role. I have found this to be counterproductive in all but the most enormous auditions. The goal is to find the best cast possible for the show. If someone seriously believes that a second attempt to sing, once the nerves are calmer, will show them to be a far better singer, it is to everyone's advantage to find out if that is true. There are limits, of course. People sometimes want to do something again or something else because they are just desperate to get your attention. Such people are usually quite obvious, and you can always decline to see them again if you think that is what is happening.

7

Rehearsals

In one sense, rehearsal is rehearsal; day in and day out the director will do much the same thing as at rehearsals for any other play, the choreographer as at any dance rehearsal, and so on. And yet there are a number of persistent problems that occur during musical rehearsals that are either different from or much more complex than in any other kinds of rehearsals. These deserve some additional attention and advice.

SCHEDULING REHEARSALS

The most frustrating aspect of musical rehearsals is that at almost no time will all the cast be present at the same time in the same place. By necessity the cast works in small groups. You may hold rehearsals every evening Monday through Friday from 7:00 to 10:00 P.M., but such rehearsals may be located in three different rooms on any given night, with some people singing in one place while others are dancing in another, and still others are working on a scene in a third. Some of the cast may work steadily for all three hours, while others may be needed for only a short half-hour session on one small part of the show; some may spend an hour with each group, and others may not be needed at all.

Such rehearsals demand precise and careful scheduling, which in turn demands detailed coordination among all three directors. As soon as the cast is known, the three directors, the stage manager, and the

128

producer (if a producer is used) must sit down and plan the *entire* rehearsal period. The planning for these rehearsals must be much more detailed and precise than for the rehearsals shown on the production schedule (see Chapter 5).

This is done after casting rather than before, so that you can take into account specific conflicts in cast schedules, if such conflicts still exist. It does you little good to plan a detailed rehearsal schedule and then have to remake it after you cast a principal singer who has evening classes every Tuesday night.

The schedule should be as exact as possible in the circumstances of a given show. Although it may seem odd to predict what you will need to rehearse four weeks from today, you can predict to a reasonable extent, and it is essential that you do. If you plan to have the show ready by a certain date, then the choreographer must know that there will be adequate rehearsal time for the dances planned (or adjust the plans to fit the rehearsal time available). The same kinds of things apply to the stage director or the music director as well; at some point, each will need to use the stage and must know ahead of time when the various spaces are available in order to plan and organize his or her own share of the rehearsals.

Detailed scheduling is simplified by the inclusion of several "worst scenes" days, usually about two weeks apart. On that day everyone in the cast is automatically scheduled (although they may be excused at the last minute), and the time is used to work on the scenes or numbers that are not developing as quickly as hoped or to make up the time lost when someone unexpectedly missed a rehearsal. With these in the schedule, you aren't forced to redo the entire schedule when something does not go according to plan.

REHEARSING

As with any form of performance, rehearsals for a musical can be broken into five basic stages. The complexity of the musical means that these five basic periods often take a far different form than for a nonmusical play, which is reflected in the way the musical rehearsal period is scheduled.

Stage 1:
Learning the Parts

In typical nonmusical rehearsals the performer is expected to learn the part on his or her own time, although a certain amount of line practice goes on in the blocking rehearsals and a certain amount of character analysis and study is discussed with the director at rehearsals.

For a musical, most of the learning of parts is actually done during the rehearsals themselves. This is simply the nature of the beast; as a result, always plan on *at least* two more weeks to rehearse a musical than a nonmusical.

There are several good reasons why musical performers cannot be left to learn their parts on their own:

1. Dance routines must be taught by rote. Each step is demonstrated by the choreographer and then repeated by the dancers until such time as the entire dance is learned. There is no other way to teach choreography. This takes time, in many cases far longer than any other aspect of the rehearsal period. In most productions the dancers may still be in the learning stage of rehearsals when other parts of the show are almost ready for final polishing.
2. Few if any of your singers will be able to read music. This means that the songs must usually be taught by rote as well, note for note, line by line. This also takes time, especially for the chorus.
3. If you work from sides, no performers will have any idea what their lines are about or even to whom they are addressed until they actually play out the scenes. In effect, they have to learn their parts by hearing the scenes in rehearsal.

Everything in the musical is keyed to the music, and thus all rehearsal periods should begin with the music, and the music rehearsals should begin with the chorus parts. In practice the chorus simply cannot function without a secure understanding of their music. For the most part they have no scripts, so that everything they do on stage will be cued in some way to the music that they sing or hear. They must know their songs before they can be blocked or rehearsed in anything else. When they dance as well, the dances will grow out of the music they sing, and even the dance rehearsals should not begin until the chorus members who also dance have grasped at least the essentials of the music. In addition they almost always work in groups, which makes everything more complicated and takes far more time than their time on stage would seem to justify. *Always* start the learning rehearsals with the chorus.

The main point of these initial rehearsals is to learn the notes and the words. Polishing and making music of them will come later. If there is any hesitancy about notes in any part of the cast, that hesitancy has a way of carrying over into every other aspect of the show. For whatever irrational reasons, every performer in the cast would rather appear on stage naked than think someone might hear them miss a note; they will mumble, twitch, and sleepwalk through scenes in terror of that one note they didn't quite learn properly in the first week of rehearsals. Take your time in these rehearsals and don't let anyone out of them until you are sure they know all the notes and words.

As soon as possible the chorus and dancers should then go to the choreographer to begin work on the dance numbers. Then and only then should the music director start work with the principals.

In my own productions I actively discourage casts from learning parts by listening to cast albums because the results are usually imitations of the recording rather than performances of the songs. Some music directors, however, find it helps people who have no musical training and no piano at home to sing along with selections. This does not work very well for chorus members; they tend to sing along with the melody while their own parts may be the harmony notes. Thus they learn the wrong music at home and have to be constantly retaught at rehearsals.

Very often the stage director will use the time when the chorus members are singing to begin discussions and possibly some rehearsal with principals. But in most essential points the first full week of rehearsals should be devoted almost exclusively to learning the music. At the end of that time the cast members should be expected to know the notes and music from memory.

Learning dialogue is a more complex issue. Unlike dance or music, lines are written down in a form all can read and therefore can be studied and memorized away from rehearsals. At the same time it is often all but impossible to rehearse some scenes without the music. Thus, the time when lines must be memorized will vary, depending on the show itself. In general, cast members should be expected to work completely from memory during the third week of rehearsals or the fourth at the latest for very complex shows.

Stage 2:
Blocking

Blocking is the working out of the significant activity and placement of the performers on the stage. It describes who stands where, does what, and when, and includes such general aspects of the performance as entrances, exits, movement in nondance sequences, and basic business.

Blocking is determined by a combination of the director's plans made prior to the beginning of rehearsals and the adjustments, inspirations, and alterations made by the director and the performers during the rehearsal period. As such, it is primarily the responsibility of the stage director, although many of the basic principles of blocking are important to the shape of the dance numbers as well.

Some directors of nonmusicals prefer to let blocking develop as the actors grow in their roles and become adjusted to the scenery and props. This is an extremely inconvenient method for a musical, however, for several reasons. First, due to the requirements of music and dance, the musical is rehearsed out of sequence; therefore, the performers have no continuity to grow in. Second, the typical musical has no set and props in the normal meaning of the term, as the typical set consists of a drop and lots of empty flat space with one or two props or furniture pieces; consequently, there is little opportunity for real interaction with those elements to help the actors develop their own blocking. As a result, when left to themselves, the performers tend to all stand as close to center as possible and do nothing. Third, the dance must grow out of the other blocking and cannot wait for such blocking to develop on its own; the choreographer cannot begin or end numbers without understanding how they are to fit into the scenes in which they are found. Everything is simplified if the director begins by dictating the blocking and then adjusts and modifies it when necessary as the show develops in rehearsals.

All blocking is immediately written down in the production book, which is the record of the entire production (see Chapter 8), as well as in the scripts of individual performers.

All blocking should be written *in pencil*. Blocking is always subject to revision. The production book is a record of the production, not Holy Writ, no matter how well the director may have planned the staging. It may be changed at any time. In addition, most musical material will be rented with the proviso that it be returned in a clean state. Every mark must be erasable.

Musical casts in particular have a tendency not to write things down in their scripts: Some are worried about ruining the rental material; others are sure they can remember such simple directions; and chorus members tend to depend on each other, each one assuming that his or her neighbor will remember so that they can just follow their neighbor through the staging. It is important to take the time to see that all blocking is written down by the performers involved, for this will save lots of time in later rehearsals. The point that so many performers and directors forget about musicals is that there may be days or even weeks between rehearsals on the same scenes. No matter how clear or obvious some direction may seem when it is given, by the time the scene is repeated hundreds of other directions will have intervened.

Most blocking for a show can and should be done in the first or second week of rehearsals. Given the nature of the musical script, it is possible to block large chunks of the show in a very short time. No one sings or dances during the blocking rehearsals, although all numbers are talked through, so that can often be done at the same time as performers are learning music, if the nature of the show allows you to block one set of characters while others are learning songs. It is usually a waste of time to block a scene with a song before the performers have at least learned the notes and words of the song. This is especially true in chorus numbers. In some unusual cases I have waited until as late as a week before opening to block a scene that included complex music or dance routines, because it took that long for dancers and singers to be secure enough in their parts to work on the scene as a whole. It is rarely wise to wait so long, but it is better to do so than to waste time trying to stage material when the cast has no idea what you are talking about.

Blocking must deal with four basic considerations: focus of attention, visualization of emotion and personal relationships, picturization in both pleasing and varied visual arrangements, and unification of style and activity for the show as a whole. Each of these topics can be studied at great length and are covered in some detail in the books on general stage direction listed in the Bibliography. However, there are some additional persistent problems in the staging of musicals that bear emphasis. In the following discussions it is assumed that you are working on a proscenium stage, for almost all successful musicals are written for such a stage.

Focus

Given a stage full of potential distractions, an audience may be tempted to look at a number of things in any given scene. One of the functions of blocking is to arrange the bodies on the stage so that the audience is encouraged to look at the person who is most important at the given moment.

In most dialogue scenes of the show focus is arranged as in any stage production, because the number of people involved is usually no more than three. Many scenes in a musical, however, involve crowds—the chorus, either staged alone or with a soloist—and this causes serious focusing problems.

The crowd (when used without soloists) is traditionally arranged in one of two ways, the line or the semicircle. These formations have the advantage of treating each character in the crowd equally and the disadvantage of being visually boring and undynamic; once the line or semicircle has been established, it makes the number look more like a choir concert than a musical production. This can be most effectively prevented by breaking the crowd into smaller groups and then arranging them so that focus can be shifted from group to group during the number, or so that individual members or entire small groups can shift and flow into other areas as the scene develops (see Picturization, page 142).

Most problems develop when the "crowd" is joined by one or more soloists. Then the problem is to focus audience attention on the soloist rather than on anyone in the crowd.

The traditional solution is to use the same lines and semicircles, but move them upstage; then the soloist steps down from the line or into the center of the semicircle. This has the advantage of simplicity and disadvantage of visual boredom if continued for any length of time. An additional disadvantage when most of the audience is at stage level is that the principal is not always visually separated from the mass of the crowd.

In order to increase separation from the mass, a follow-spot is added to focus on a principal performer and follow him or her around the stage. This focuses attention on the soloist.

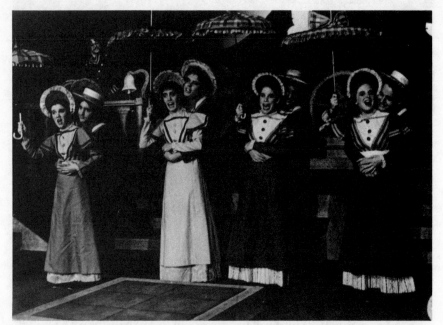

FIGURE 10. Equal Focus in a Line. Typical chorus arrangement stressing each person equally. *H.M.S. Pinafore*, College of Notre Dame, Belmont, CA. Directed by Robert Titlow. Photo courtesy College of Notre Dame.

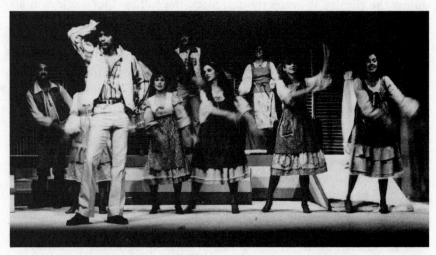

FIGURE 11. Focus Against a Line. Soloist stands downstage of chorus arranged in lines above. *Two Gentlemen of Verona*, Bakersfield Community Theatre, Bakersfield, CA. Direction and photo by David Grote.

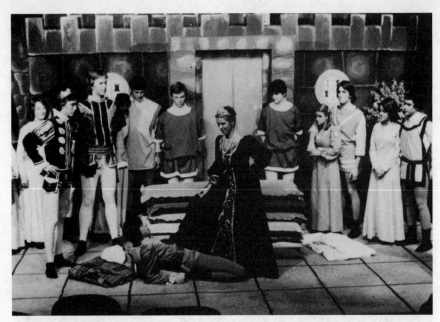

FIGURE 12. Focus Against a Semicircle. Chorus forms semicircle and soloists play in imaginary center point of circle. *Once Upon a Mattress*, De Smet Jesuit High School, St. Louis, MO. Directed and designed by John Faust. Photo courtesy John Faust.

There are occasionally some practical technical reasons why this must be done (see Chapter 8), but it rarely solves the problem. First, unless the theatre is perfectly designed, the follow-spot angle will always be too low, which throws the same light on the parts of the crowd directly behind the soloist, the very people who need to be most clearly separated from the soloist. Second, the difference in intensity between follow-spot and other lighting often demands different makeup for the people who must work in the spot and sometimes causes serious adjustment problems for the eyes of the audience as they shift from spotlighted scenes to regular lighted scenes. Third, decisions about who should be in the spot often lead to serious conflict among the performers because those not spotlighted in effect disappear from the audience view. Finally, even if the follow-spot tries to move from person to person as needed, the movement of the light itself soon becomes so distracting that all sense of the scene itself is lost.

There are other ways to handle the problem of focusing on a soloist in relation to the group. Some of these include the following:

1. Focusing by variation The soloist takes a different piece of business or activity; for example, the soloist stands while the crowd sits, or sits

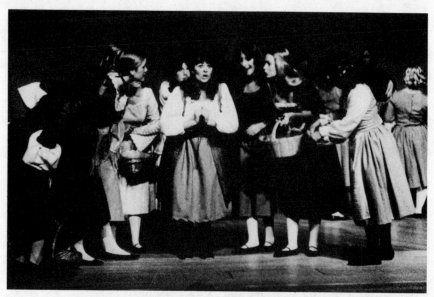

FIGURE 13. Focus Against Semicircle. Tight semicircle makes soloist part of the group while still separated as soloist. Note also use of lighter costume colors to visually separate soloist from group. *Brigadoon*, Highland High School, Bakersfield, CA. Directed and designed by Susan Archibald Grote. Photo by David Grote.

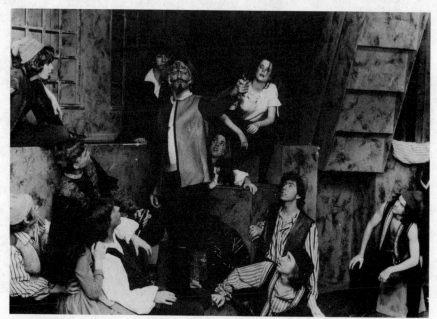

FIGURE 14. Focus by Variation. Soloist stands while other characters kneel or sit. *Man of La Mancha*, De Smet Jesuit High School, St. Louis, MO. Directed and designed by John Faust. Photo courtesy John Faust.

while the crowd stands, moves to the left while the group moves right, moves while the crowd is still, and so on.

2. Focusing by separation The soloist is visually separated from the crowd, to one side or on a different scenic level, or by a unique, eye-catching costume.

3. Focusing by triangulation The group is arranged in a rough triangle on the stage, and the soloist is placed at one of the points, or the group is arranged as two sides of a triangle with the soloist alone on the third side. This is especially effective when focus must shift several times in close succession; by simply changing the direction in which the crowd looks, focus will change to a different point or side of the triangle without having to move the bodies around.

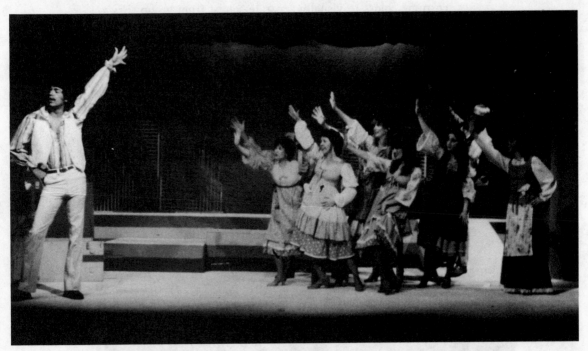

FIGURE 15. Focus by Separation. Soloist at opposite side of stage from chorus. *Two Gentlemen of Verona*, Bakersfield Community Theatre, Bakersfield, CA. Direction and photo by David Grote.

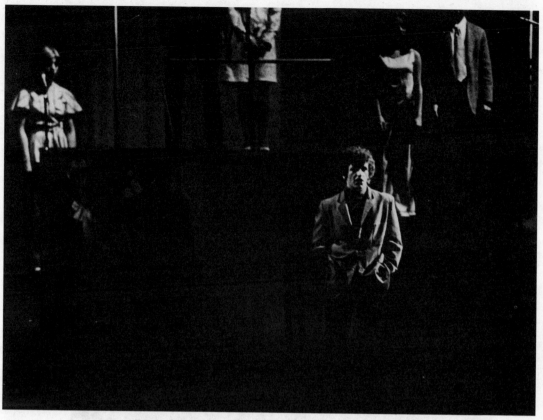

FIGURE 16. Focus by Separation. Soloist plays on a different scenic level from rest of chorus. Note also use of variable lighting levels to separate soloist from chorus members on same level, without follow-spot. *Company*, South High School, Bakersfield, CA. Direction, design, and photo by David Grote.

Numerous additional examples and suggestions may be found in the books listed in the Bibliography related to directing or choreography.

When planning focus, remember that a photograph shows only a still moment, while the musical is constantly in motion. None of the many different focusing methods will work if it is the only method used in the show or if it is used unvaryingly through a single number. Good blocking and choreography continually adjusts and modifies focus, using many different methods as needed to provide an interesting whole.

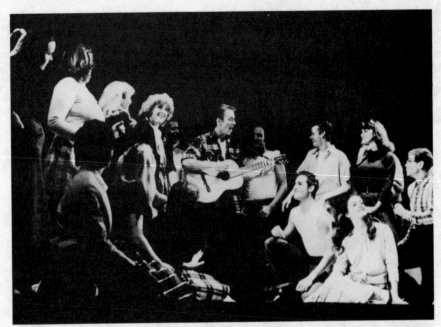

FIGURE 17. Focus by Triangle. Soloist at upstage point of triangle. *Grease*, Theatre Concord, Concord, CA. Directed by Patrick Payton, designed by Jeffrey Rowlings, costumes by Sheila Viramontes, photo by Theatrix. Photo courtesy Scott Quintard.

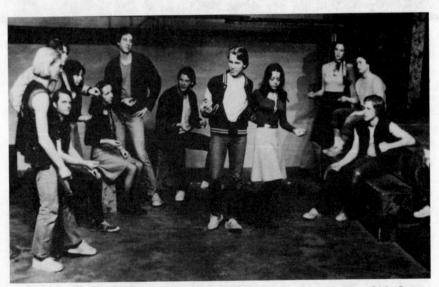

FIGURE 18. Focus by Triangle. Soloists in center of triangle. *West Side Story*, De Smet Jesuit High School, St. Louis, MO. Directed and designed by John Faust. Photo courtesy John Faust.

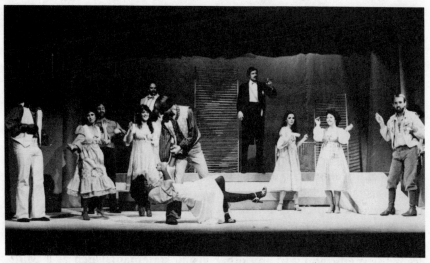

FIGURE 19. Focus by Triangle. Soloists on one side of triangle, chorus on other two sides. *Two Gentlemen of Verona*, Bakersfield Community Theatre, Bakersfield, CA. Direction and photo by David Grote.

Visualization

The blocking of the show should make visible the emotions of the characters involved. In general, this is done through the development of specific physical business that demonstrates how the character feels about each line and each situation. The plotting of the actual moves from one part of the stage to another is the responsibility of the director, while all other business is the responsibility of the performer and the director working together.

There are no specific rules for this part of the blocking, as each character and each performer must express themselves in different ways. The important point to remember, however, is that the script describes a process of change. Each change of emotions should be mirrored visually. Some of these changes may be large, while others are very delicate and small, but no change in emotion should ever go by without a corresponding change in some visual aspect of the staging.

In addition, the blocking should demonstrate visually the relationships between the characters and any changes in those relationships. This is relatively easy when several people or large groups are

141

on stage, but it is often difficult when you must deal with a solo or a duet scene or song.

Picturization

The blocking should be arranged in a way that is visually interesting. This is usually called picturization. In general, the proscenium of the stage serves as a picture frame, within which the scenery and the performers must be arranged to make an interesting visual composition. This requires some sense of balance and artistic composition in each scene, as might apply to any other visual statement, such as a painting or a photograph.

However, the "rules" for such compositions are in effect more difficult to apply on the stage, because gravity keeps all the people at the bottom of the frame (on the stage floor), where they would never be in a painting. In addition, few people in the audience will be at ideal viewing positions; what is balanced and attractive to someone seated in the twelfth-row center may be incomprehensible to someone in the first row on the side or someone else in the front of the balcony. Thus, the rules suggested in many directing and design books must always be adjusted to fit a particular situation on your own stage and modified through your own eyes.

More important for the show as a whole is the need for variety. Each moment should look somewhat different from every other moment. This is especially difficult to achieve with musicals, which concentrate on the two hardest kinds of scenes to vary—the crowd scene and the solo.

The key to working with crowd scenes is to remember that the crowd is composed of a group of individuals. Even when identified only as "chorus," they are characters who serve some dramatic function, no matter how minimal, and thus must be staged as individuals, not in lumps. Once you begin to work in this way, the ways in which the group can be arranged are expanded enormously. This requires a lot of what is often referred to as "traffic direction"—detailed attention to individuals to keep them moving in various ways without running into each other.

In particular, remember that *the chorus is allowed to move*. This often comes as a shock to both music directors and singers, who are used to standing still in order to concentrate on the singing. But the chorus cannot be allowed to do this in a musical. The movement must be purposeful; it is not movement for movement's sake. The singers can and should move, both to visualize their relationships and to vary the stage picture.

With solos the problem seems more pronounced. How can you produce variety with only one person? The key to this is to remember that each song or monologue deals with a unique, specific situation. The song may be expository, but the information in that exposition must be made visible in some way that is different for each song. Even when the primary information is personal emotion, the revelation of that feeling costs the character something, and the effort it takes for the character to make that revelation is what should be staged. The "problem" often disappears when you stop thinking "turn left, sit down, stand," and so forth and start thinking about the content of the specific song.

Variety is also required in use of the space. Musicals tend to be heavily center-weighted: scenes with only one or two people naturally gravitate to the center of the stage (to down center in particular), which is both a strong visual position and one close to the microphones. Large scenes, unless carefully developed, tend to scatter the crowd around various parts of the stage above and to the side while leaving principals and soloists standing at center or down center. As a result, it is possible for some characters to go through an entire show without ever moving more than a step or two in any direction from the down-center position except to exit completely from the stage. Needless to say this can quickly become boring. Wherever possible try to "save" the strong down-center position for the most important and dramatic moments in the show and move the principals around the whole stage space at various times during the show.

Picturization in the musical is complicated by one further unique problem: The characters sing with and over an accompaniment. Thus, they *must* be able to face the audience at all times when they are speaking or singing. It is relatively common in nonmusicals to have some people face across the stage or even upstage much of the time, but in musicals this should be done sparingly, and never during the actual singing of a song. Performers have to aim sound outward to compete with the orchestra or the piano. Audiences have to be able to

read lips to help them understand lyrics in songs. If there are microphones, the performers must speak consistently within the patterns of
the microphones, which means that even in dialogue scenes they cannot turn very far toward the wings or their voices will drop below the
sound level to which the audience has become adjusted. This often
results in some odd poses, such as the man standing behind the woman
and singing into her ear rather than looking into her eyes during a romantic duet, but that is part of the form. This severely limits some of
the ways you can arrange the stage picture and vary the groupings in
a scene.

Finally, use your strongest parts of the stage and your most dramatic stage pictures for the most important parts of the show. Each
scene has a small climax, usually at the end of the last song in that

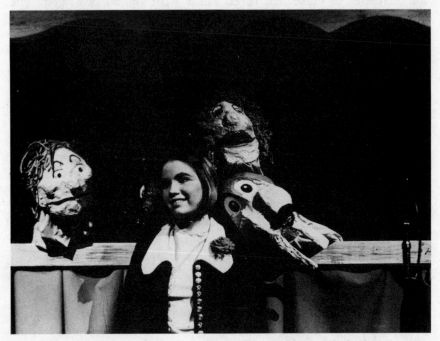

FIGURE 20. Playing to Audience. Actress is speaking and singing to puppets, but does not face them; rather, she faces out, a typical artificial arrangement necessary to keep sound aimed out to
microphones and audience. *Carnival!*, South High School,
Bakersfield, CA. Puppets by Joanne Thomas, direction, design, and photo by David Grote.

scene. The first act has a somewhat larger climax just before the intermission, and the show as a whole has a major climax in the last act. Save your strongest places and your great stage pictures for those points in the production. And whatever you do, even with solos, don't march the singers down in front of a microphone to stand stock-still throughout the song. Frank Sinatra can sell a song while simply standing in front of a microphone, but not many in your cast are Sinatras; the performers must be staged so as to exploit the dramatic as well as the musical elements in each song.

Unification

Each show and each production has its own style of presentation, which should be developed in all aspects of the production. In the planning stages of the show you will have agreed on a style for your production, to be followed in your choice of the scenery, costumes, lighting, and so on. It is essential that this stylistic decision be carried through in the blocking of the show as well. Certain kinds of business, certain kinds of stage pictures, and certain patterns of movement can be used in a show while certain others are out of place, no matter how momentarily funny or attractive they might be.

It is especially important in this consideration that the blocking of the show as a whole coordinate with the kind of patterns and attitudes to be expressed in the dances of the show. Not only must the blocking put the dancers in position to begin their numbers, but it must also establish the stylistic mood and statement from which such numbers can grow out of the show as a whole, so they appear to belong to a unified production rather than seeming simply stuck in at random.

Finally, the unification of the blocking must lead the audience through the show toward the climax. In this way certain key points in the plot development are indicated in the staging so that the audience recognizes them as such. Always remember that this is a dramatic production, not just a succession of musical numbers. The show as a whole must both fit together and move toward an emotional climax of some kind.

Stage 3:
Development

The development period is the meat of the rehearsal. Surprisingly, however, this is the part of the rehearsal most amateur groups tend to skip over. There is a tendency among not only amateur performers but also among directors who work with them to think that such groups are good only by accident. If they get all the words right, stay together in the dances, and don't trip over anything in performance, then they are thought to have done as well as they can. Performers who are allowed to believe this spend all their rehearsal period learning their parts and never thinking about anything else. The result is a typical "amateur" production. But if the development sequence in the rehearsals is used seriously, then the show can be good by any standards, not just good to the parents and relatives in the audience.

The key to a good development period is to demand that it be used for genuine role development, not more fumbling on lines and notes. No matter what individual performers may claim, they cannot think in depth about the role if they are trying to remember the words, notes, or dance steps. Nor can any other people who work with them in scenes, even if they know their parts well already; the people who know their parts must constantly worry about what the others may do at any moment, with the result that little real growth occurs in the rehearsal. Leave adequate time in the learning stage of rehearsals for parts to be learned, but then be adamant that the learning period must end, so that *real* rehearsals can begin.

During the development period each of the three directors takes every scene and number apart in detail, trying to shape each moment into the best possible expression of that moment for the show as a whole. Music directors will work on every song in detail, trying to produce the best sound, the best phrasing, the best dramatic expression for each song, and then fit that into the blocking developed for the song by the stage director and the actor. The choreographer will try to turn the set of steps into a sequence of a dance, a unit that flows from beginning to end. The stage director will work with every scene, trying to develop specific characters and emotional lines, focus jokes, establish relationships between the characters, and make dramatic sense of each word in the show, *including the lyrics of the songs*. In addition, the stage director must be able to adjust the blocking as required by new ideas and insights, problems the music director raises about the needs of the singers, and technical problems that become known as the rehearsals progress.

One of the most easily overlooked aspects of these rehearsals is the development of specific characters for each of the chorus members. How can you dramatically justify the sudden appearance of a crowd where moments before the stage was empty? How can you make this look both logical and effortless? This requires not only practical planning, such as the careful placement of all chorus members in the wings before their entrance so they don't bump into the scenery or each other while coming on or going off; it also requires dramatic planning so that each chorus member has just as much individual reason and purpose for coming into the scene as any of the principals would have.

There is no one best way to rehearse performers, and even if there were a work of this size could not hope to explain it. For those looking for ways to expand their repertoire of rehearsal techniques, however, a number of the works listed in the Bibliography will be quite valuable. The following practical points may help as well.

It is usually best for the music director to begin detailed work in the development period with the principals. They must integrate their songs into the dialogue scenes far more extensively than the chorus and thus need to polish their songs much sooner in order to rehearse their other scenes seriously. While the principals work with the music, the stage director and the choreographer can devote detailed attention to the chorus members, staging their scenes, developing their basic characterizations, and working on dance numbers in which they figure.

During this period nothing should be rehearsed in units larger than a single scene. There is no practical way that scenes can be rehearsed in sequence unless there are simultaneous music/dance/scene rehearsals, so don't waste time trying to start at the beginning. Time can be used much more efficiently and effectively by arranging rehearsals in short scenes and then having each director see several different scenes on a single evening.

In general, it is better to spend no more than an hour at a time on any single scene or song at any one rehearsal, unless that scene is uniquely long and complex like the assembly scenes in *1776*. If a scene needs three hours of serious work, it is usually better to do it in three separate sessions—for one simple reason. No matter how well performers do a scene in one rehearsal, they will forget some of what they did the next time that scene is rehearsed. The longer they have between repetitions of that scene, the more they will forget. Thus if it is at all possible, plan your schedule so that you never wait more than a week before repeating or restudying a particular scene during the development period. This may be only a quick fifteen-minute review just to keep a good scene looking good, but such review is essential, even with experienced casts.

Once singers have learned and then studied the songs, they should sing them in scene rehearsals. The scenes cannot grow dramatically if the performers skip the most dramatic parts of the scenes—the songs that begin or end them. At this time, while the music director and the accompanist are still working with other singers, it helps to have the accompanist make a practice tape for the stage director to use during scene rehearsals.

Stage 4:
Integration

Once the small pieces of the show have been developed in detail, the various pieces must be put together into a show. This occurs in three different steps of integration:

1. music and dance into scenes
2. scenes into sequence
3. technical integration into performance

At integration rehearsals all three directors should be present at all times, for several important reasons. As music and dance are integrated into scenes, then into a sequence, and so on, adjustments will have to be made in the staging, choreography, and even in some musical aspects. Such changes require the participation of all the directors, if for no other reason than to avoid giving contradictory directions. In addition, when performers are faced with anything new, they tend to forget part of something they seemed to know perfectly well. For example, without the music director present to remind the singers how to support the sound, they tend to forget to do so when trying to find their entrance among new scenery pieces. In the same way dancers will forget to extend a motion completely or actors will drop pieces of business or blocking while trying to cope with *all* the various things they have to remember in these very complex rehearsals. Thus all directors, not just the stage director, must be present at these rehearsals.

Scene integration

A certain amount of integration begins during the development rehearsals, of course, particularly for principals who sing in short scenes. But the integration period is devoted to the complete integration of material with the full emotional and physical intensity of the performance.

If the development rehearsals have been detailed and intensive, this stage will be very brief. It is devoted mostly to familiarizing the various people with those parts of the show they were not directly involved in, so that the principals learn to work with the chorus, chorus learns how they fit into specific scenes, and so on. If you have tried to skimp on the development period, however, this will be a long and trying period.

This is a particularly complex stage in the rehearsals for chorus members and dancers. Most of them have not yet grasped quite how their songs or dances fit into the scenes, and there will be many reminders and adjustments before they find all their places and begin to start "acting" through the scene as a whole. In many cases principals will have rarely sung or performed with the chorus, rehearsing in different places at different times, and there must be a certain amount of coordination and familiarization.

Rehearsals in this period deal with one scene at a time, with no particular attempt to establish a sequence.

Sequential integration

The next step is to fit each of the completed scenes into a sequence. This normally produces two quite different kinds of problems.

First, you must solve the physical problems of simply moving through the show as a whole. These tend to be extensive. Singers suddenly find that where they thought they had ten minutes between songs, they really have only five. People who always exited vigorously into the empty wings at the end of one scene suddenly discover that the wings are full of people waiting to come on for the next scene, so that there is nowhere to go. Some of the cast will even forget what scenes come next at any given moment or what scene they are in when they come on stage. For a few days it may seem to the directors as if the show is going backward, but this should sort itself out quickly if the stage director and stage manager respond to problem areas with quick solutions.

The emotional problems are even more critical, for this is when the performers must shape their roles *as a whole*. Because the nature of the musical makes run-throughs of sequences or of the whole show all but impossible before this time, the performers will have only theoretical experience with the totality of their roles or of the show. In the development period, cast and directors worked on tiny details while trying to keep the whole performance in mind, but it takes a lot of time and work to shape that whole performance, no matter how detailed the work might have been. During this period the stage director must modify and adjust the rhythm and the visual shape of the show to make the script dramatically clear. The cast must establish continuity and growth for their characters. This stage should normally take about a week of rehearsals and cannot be successfully accomplished in one quick run-through, as so many groups try to do.

The last rehearsal before you begin technical integration should be a full run-through of the show with the rehearsal accompanist, and it should be at performance intensity. If the show is going to look good, it will look good at this rehearsal. If this rehearsal looks bad, you have very little time to salvage the show. In a very real sense, this is your opening night and the date toward which you should aim all your rehearsals. After this point, technical problems will occupy everyone's attention, and there will be little time or energy to improve or change any parts of the performances themselves. If the performers aren't ready, they will have little opportunity in the next week to get any better.

Technical integration

There are two different aspects to technical integration for a musical. One is the integration of the orchestra with the singers and dancers. If at all possible, this step should not be taken at the same time as other technical integration. An orchestra and a piano sound completely different. No matter how well the performers have been rehearsed, and no matter how good the orchestra might be, the first rehearsal with the orchestra is a shock; no one will be able to find their notes, know which instruments to follow, if any, or recognize their cues. Thus it is best for singers to have at least one rehearsal in which they do nothing but sing with the orchestra before trying to work with the orchestra in the context of the complete show. This will ultimately save an enormous amount of pain and time in other rehearsals when the performers should be polishing the show, not trying to find their notes.

The second area is far more complex: the integration of all scenery, costumes, lights, sound, props, and so on, into the established sequence of the show. This occurs during what are called the technical or tech rehearsals.

In an ideal world where you make your own scenery and costumes and control your own stage, the cast should begin to rehearse with these items as soon as they are available. Dancers should rehearse in their costumes, blocking should be done in front of scenery pieces or with the real furniture, and so on. In that way the cast and directors face no surprises at the last minute, and problems can be solved under considerably less pressure.

Unfortunately, such an ideal world is very rare. For the most part, major portions of your technical elements will be rented and will not arrive until about a week before opening night. In many cases, if you rent a stage, you will not be able to move in on that stage for rehearsals or to install your technical equipment until about a week before you open. Even when you build or control your own stage, the schedule might not allow you to finish most of the items until the last week of the show. In such cases you must try to make the best of things and install and adjust the technical aspects of your show as efficiently and as quickly as possible.

Many groups try to do this all at once in gigantic twelve-to-fifteen-hour sessions on the Saturday and Sunday before the show opens.

In most cases this is not only counterproductive but disastrous. Many a muscle has been pulled, many a vocal cord destroyed, and many a nerve frayed beyond repair in such sessions, and the casts are left so completely exhausted that the show never recovers and a few of the cast swear never to be in another show again in their lives. This need not happen in a properly organized situation. When faced with these Saturday/Sunday messes, I have found that the following general approach seems to work best:

1. As early as possible on Saturday, the stage and light crews install the scenery and lights under the supervision of the TD and/or the designers.

2. During the morning, but after the heavy crews have had a chance to get the bulky items out of the way, the prop crew moves in furniture and props.

3. At about the same time, the costume crew begins fitting performers into any of the rented costumes that have not yet been fitted. All locally made costumes should have been fitted long before this time, and if it is possible to get rented costumes sooner, then they should have been fitted as well. As soon as this is done, the performers should help the other crews install their equipment on stage.

4. By the middle of the afternoon the lighting crew should be able to begin setting the cues. The set crew must change scenery for the light crew because cues cannot be set without scenery pieces in their proper place. The stage manager can then use this same period to organize the scene changes.

5. In early evening, the entire cast should arrive and dress for the show but without makeup. All crews, designers, and directors should also be called for this rehearsal.

6. When everyone is ready, walk through the show. In a walk-through rehearsal, the performers go through all their business, handle all the props, practice all the entrances and exits, make all their costume changes, and go through all their blocking without speaking lines or singing, or with only enough of such to remind them where they are. If there are obvious problems with something the performers must deal with, stop and solve the problem. At each entrance or change of position on stage, check the lighting, practice sound effects, and so on, and make notes of anything that needs to be changed. But if the change requires a significant amount of time, don't stop to fix it at this point. There is no excuse for any re-

hearsal in which performers must stand around on stage for half an hour at a time while the light crew tries to set light cues for a number or for them to repeat an entrance a dozen times while the stage manager tries to get the scene change organized. This will be a long rehearsal, no matter how well organized it is, so don't make it worse than it needs to be.

7. When you reach the end of the walkthrough, each director, designer, and crew head will have a long list of things that need to be fixed or corrected. Send the cast home, have a quick production meeting, and decide or agree what is to be done about the various problems.

8. As early as possible or necessary on Sunday morning, the crews come back to modify the lighting, practice scene changes, adjust the costumes, and so on.

9. At this time the sound man can begin to install the microphones and other sound reinforcement equipment for the production. In general, trying to install the sound equipment at the same time as the set pieces will only result in extra confusion. If the scenery and lights are installed first, then the sound man can usually set up very quickly and test the results in that evening's rehearsal.

10. In the middle of the afternoon the cast should be called again for a complete run-through of the show, with full acting, singing, and dancing. Every effort should be made to go without stopping, but if there are still problems that the actors need to have solved, stop and solve them. If there are problems the designers wish to solve, such as additional modifications of the lighting or other problems that do not directly affect the actors, wait until the evening when the actors can be released. In this way you get the maximum work accomplished with the minimum drain on company energy, resources, and nerves.

If at all possible, try to avoid putting your tech rehearsals at such a late date. The more technical rehearsals you can have, the better the show will look and the calmer the performers will be. A technical rehearsal is like a dress rehearsal with one difference; you may stop during the tech rehearsal to solve a problem. Dress rehearsals have a different function, which will be discussed in stage 5.

Generally the orchestra is added at the last tech rehearsal. By that time most of the other technical problems should have been dealt with, so that all attention can be focused on timing the music, getting accustomed to the cues from the orchestra and the conductor, and adjusting the sound system to deal with the orchestra as well as the performers on stage.

One of the most important rules I have learned through painful experience is that *the cast should never face more than one new thing at a time*; that is, they should concentrate on costumes for the first time in a rehearsal other than the ones in which they first work with real props or with the orchestra. They should never have to cope with all the technical aspects of the show at the same rehearsal unless there is simply no other way to do things.

Stage 5: Polishing

The last part of the rehearsal period is devoted to dress rehearsals. A dress rehearsal is just like a performance with one difference—no audience is present. The purpose of the dress rehearsals is to polish the show, to give it that little extra zing and sparkle that makes a show special.

Many people look for tricks that will spark up a show at the last minute, but there really is rarely any need of tricks. The most important factor in polishing a show is the performers' sense of security in the show. If they have been carefully rehearsed, if they know what they need to do, know how to do it, and *know that they know how to do it,* then they can concentrate on doing it. Too many performers spend most of their time on stage trying to remember what to do next or worrying that what is supposed to happen will not happen. They worry whether the lights will come on, whether they will find their note for the song, whether the other people on stage will finally say all the lines they're supposed to say, whether the cup will have coffee in it, or hundreds of other distracting things. If they didn't have to worry about such things, they could concentrate on playing the role, on saying and doing what the characters do. This is the first and foremost function of the dress rehearsal. Before an audience sees the show, the cast and crews all go through it a few times so that they really believe they can do it the same way all the time. If they in fact can do this, then when the audience is added, the cast will really take off and you will have a good show.

Of course, the performers don't become secure in their performance if the dress rehearsals are fiascos or if they are really tech rehearsals, with constant stopping and starting to fix this or that, or with scenery and props that still don't work, or lights that are constantly being adjusted while they try to perform. These things should be done during tech rehearsals, but if there are still problems, call special rehearsals for the crews or the individual performers involved before or after the dress rehearsals themselves. Use the dress rehearsal for one thing only—establishing the flow of a complete, genuine performance.

There will still be many things to correct and adjust during the dress rehearsals. Each director should observe and make notes of problems and mistakes. Then, after the rehearsal is finished, the cast and crew heads should gather with the directors for a period of notes.

These notes should be brief. They should deal primarily with points about which the cast needs to be reminded, not things that should be completely redone. The world is full of stories about Broadway shows that were saved by major rewrites or restaging of scenes the night before opening, but none that I've been able to substantiate. In my experience, especially with amateur casts, you make major changes during tech or dress rehearsals only at great risk to the show, even when the change is designed to help the actors.

For the most part, notes should contain items like: "You still need to be a little louder in this song"; "Don't talk so fast on that punch line, or you won't get the laugh we need"; or "Remember to turn to the right when you enter—you've done that every night but tonight, so don't change it now." If more than a note is needed—if more rehearsal is necessary or a complex situation demands attention—set up a time before the next day's rehearsal to meet with the persons involved. Don't keep the whole cast around waiting to solve one person's problem. Remember that you are dealing with people who have spouses, families, and jobs that they have to go to the next morning. These obligations put an emotional and physical limit on rehearsals, even dress rehearsals. After a certain time of night, no one will hear or remember anything that is said. There are no last-minute ideas that will save the show; it was saved or lost two weeks before dress rehearsals ever began.

A note about mythology: in spite of what many believe, a bad final dress rehearsal means a bad opening night. Performances may be better than the dress rehearsal, but they will not be good unless the entire rehearsal period has made them good. When most people talk about how much better the show got after dress rehearsals, they tend to remember the last show, not the first one. *People pay the same money for the first night as for the last*; they should see just as good a show for their money.

TYPICAL PROBLEMS

"Stars"

People who are cast in major roles of a musical tend to regard themselves as something special. These roles were often played by stars in New York; therefore, whoever plays them anywhere else must also be a star, if only in the local community. This misinterprets the role of the star. Stars are not stars by virtue of their skills (although some stars do have unusual skills); stars are stars because people will pay money to see them *no matter what they are in*. Thus, as much as possible, a professional production will cater to the star's wishes, because a real star guarantees ticket buyers. At the local level, however, *everyone* is a "star." The little girl who stands at the back of the chorus in the high school show or the insurance salesman who says only two lines in the community theatre production both have just as many relatives, just as many business acquaintances, and just as many friends as the person singing the lead, and will attract just as many people to the audience. Thus, there is no justification whatsoever for treating the people with larger roles any differently from anyone else in the show.

(If anyone must be treated carefully, it should be the people in the smaller roles. If a lead role player walks off, you will have dozens of people eager to replace him or her, but you will spend days trying to find replacements if one of the players of a smaller role leaves.)

Cast Changes

In most shows, at some time during rehearsals you will have to replace part of the cast. Most changes result when performers take themselves out of the cast in some way. In all my productions where I have made cast changes, only once did I "fire" an actor; in all others, people left the cast because they got sick, had accidents, took new jobs or left town, or, if students, got punished by their parents for something completely unrelated to the show. This is why you should always begin rehearsals with an alternate cast in mind (see Chapter 6).

Much more difficult to cope with, however, are cast attendance problems that may not lead to cast changes. This usually arises from illness. If someone becomes sick, how long can you wait before you make a replacement? How do you rehearse while this person is ill and can't be at rehearsals? There is no easy answer to this. You simply must be as flexible as possible when such situations arise. Adjust rehearsal schedules to work around illnesses, keep your eye on various possibilities, and accept it as part of the process.

Much more frustrating is a cast in which a different person is missing at each rehearsal. On Tuesday someone has a cold, on Wednesday someone else has to take their son to the emergency room for a broken arm, on Thursday someone else's boss demands a report at the last minute. Such excuses are justifiable, or at least unavoidable, and there is nothing you can do to prevent them. At the same time it is terribly frustrating to realize during the fifth week of rehearsals that you have never had a rehearsal in which every person who was supposed to be on stage had actually been there. The only thing you can do is stress for the cast how important it is to everyone that they all be at all scheduled rehearsals. Remind them that when they miss one rehearsal, they in effect lose *three*—the one they miss, the one they have to use to make up the one they missed, and the one that was lost when its rehearsal was replaced by the makeup rehearsal. And everyone in the scene, even those who are there, misses these three rehearsals with every absence.

At some time it may seem necessary to replace a performer who is attending regularly. This is always a delicate area, even more so among volunteers and amateurs. The only valid reason for doing so, however, is rampant irresponsibility. People who are continually late, who are persistently unprepared, who disappear during rehearsals, who constantly talk or make trouble backstage while others are rehearsing—such people should be removed as soon as it is clear that they refuse to change their behavior. Make it clear that such behavior will not be tolerated, and if the behavior continues, replace the performer, *no matter what size of role is involved.* In the long run things will work out better than if you had kept the troublemakers around.

It is not nearly so valid to replace someone who "can't play the part." For one thing, if you had someone who could play it better, you would have cast them to begin with, wouldn't you? People try out for shows because they want to do parts and because they want to learn how to do the things that go along with that. You cannot expect them to be perfect from the first day. All the directors should expect to spend a lot of time teaching people to sing or dance or act better, or even to sing, dance, or act from scratch; it just comes with the territory anywhere outside the New York talent pool.

Prompters

A prompter is a person who follows the script during rehearsals and/ or performance and gives lines to performers on stage when they forget them.

Prompting is one of the stage manager's primary functions during rehearsals. From the moment when the performers are "off book," that is, working from memory without scripts or scores in their hands, they will have moments when they either do not remember what comes next or remember something inaccurately. Since the stage manager is at rehearsal following the production book and noting changes made by the director, he or she must naturally follow the lines and will serve as a prompter.

There is a simple and effective procedure to be used. The prompter does not give a line in rehearsal until it is asked for. When the performer forgets the next line, he or she should be instructed to freeze and say: "Line." Then the prompter reads loudly and clearly the first six to ten words of the line, at which point the performer should recognize it and go on. As long as the performer does not ask for the line, the prompter should assume that he or she will find it.

In general, the prompter should not correct a line when the performers have not stopped unless the misstatement has the wrong sense or comes from a completely different scene. The only exception would be when the director is working on an intricate scene of some sort and specifically instructs the prompter to interrupt immediately when anything is inaccurate. When performers miss a specific word or two, the stage manager/prompter should note it and then correct the performer at a pause in rehearsal before the same sequence is repeated or at the end of the rehearsal.

In my own productions, it is understood that once the stage manager must go backstage to manage the production, there will be no prompter. As Dr. Johnson said about hanging, this concentrates the mind wonderfully. Other directors feel a prompter is sometimes helpful, but in none of my productions has it ever been necessary. If someone drops a line during a show that has been well rehearsed, someone else on stage will be able to adjust, and the scene will continue smoothly, more smoothly than if everyone waits while the prompter tries to decide if the actor is *really* lost or while ghostly voices float out from the wings or the pit with the missing line.

The one advantage musicals have in this regard is that there is a visible person in the pit whose presence is already accepted by the audience—the conductor. If someone gets lost in one of the songs, the conductor is in a much better position to mouth the line for the singers and get them back in place than would be a prompter in the wings. If things break down completely and the situation is desperate, the conductor can always get out of the scene by starting the next number, although I have never done a show in which this happened. Orchestra conductors should not be prompters—they have plenty to do without those duties—but they do provide a last line of defense.

In general, line problems occur for two reasons. The first is that the lines were never learned or understood properly, which can be prevented by careful rehearsal in both the learning and the development period. The second comes simply through lack of concentration on stage by the performers themselves. This can be prevented by a constant emphasis on real concentration during rehearsals and by the tension caused by the performance itself. Very few amateur productions will run for so long that the cast has a chance to take themselves for granted; with only two or three performances a week for only a few weeks, they should have no excuse for losing their concentration enough to lose their lines in performance. Working without a prompter helps them maintain that concentration. To some people it's like a trapeze act working without a net, but in my own experience it has not only never been a problem but has usually helped the performances.

Rehearsal Environment

Rehearsals need not all take place on stage, but they should always take place in rooms that are at least as large as the stage on which the show will be performed. Without such space, the performers cannot successfully retain their blocking and choreography, nor can any of the directors see and hear rehearsals from the necessary distance.

Dance rehearsals should always be held on a real wooden floor, not on concrete or on tile or wood laid over concrete just for looks. The dancers will spend an enormous amount of time slamming their feet and legs onto the floor, and they can do serious damage to themselves if the floor has no resiliency. It should be obvious that no rehearsal hall, especially for dancers, should be carpeted; no stage will be carpeted, and no movement can be rehearsed properly when the floor is so completely different from the final performing space.

Rehearsal rooms should not be the same spaces as those used for scenery construction for obvious safety reasons. It never hurts if these rooms are also attractive and comfortable. There is a certain glamor among the uninitiated about rehearsing and working in drafty old halls among sawdust and falling ladders, but that glamor quickly wears off. When the typical unheated (or uncooled) rehearsal room, with no functioning toilets, no offstage space, and dirt and grime everywhere, is contrasted with the comparative comforts of home, it's a wonder that many groups ever find a cast at all.

Attitudes

The single most important thing that all three directors must provide during rehearsals is a good attitude toward the production. This involves keeping up a good spirit, always treating cast members positively when problems arise, and dealing with rehearsals and the inevitable crises in as levelheaded a manner as possible. Temper tantrums and absent-minded professorism make nice scenes in the movies, but they have no place in real rehearsals.

A good attitude also involves the careful control of time. No one likes to waste time. Cast members expect a certain amount of social interaction from the rehearsals, but they also expect their time to be well used because they all have other things to do with their time. The directors must know the schedule, use the schedule well, and always give the appearance of being organized. In particular they must start and end all rehearsals *exactly* as scheduled. In turn this sense of organization will rub off on the cast as a whole, and they will be more businesslike and intense in their own use of the rehearsal time.

At the same time, you must establish from the very beginning what you mean by quality work. Amateur casts will generally be as good as directors expect and allow them to be. They learn your criteria not from what you say but from what you do, by the care and seriousness with which you rehearse. If you are serious about doing the show well, they eventually will be too. If you are flighty, disorganized, artsy, or excessively casual, they will respond to that and produce flighty, disorganized, artsy, or casual performances. The directors can only push or pull a cast to the limits of their talents, but those limits are often far broader and finer than many people expect. The cast goes through rehearsal for pleasure, but that pleasure is greatest when the work is genuinely well done.

8
Technical Problems

All theatrical productions share the same potential technical problems, things like scenery, costumes, and lighting, which require the use of specialists or far more detailed instruction for beginners than can be given in the space available here. If such parts of production are new to you or the members of your organization, refer to the books in the Bibliography. However, even for experienced workers, there are some persistent problems that are, for the most part, unique to musicals, which we can briefly examine here.

DROPS

The scenery item most typical of the musical and the item most often rented and thus not available for practice sessions is the drop. This large flat piece of canvas or other heavy-duty material is generally a little wider and taller than the opening in your proscenium. It is called a drop because when it is not in use it is pulled up out of sight into the space above the stage, from which it is then dropped down when needed for use.

A full set of drops for a show will consist of several different kinds. The most crucial is the full-stage drop, often called a back drop because it covers the entire width of the stage and hangs at the back of the scene for which it serves as scenery. These full-stage drops can hang far upstage, or they can serve as the drops for scenes-in-one or -in-two (see Chapter 3). In most shows, these full stage drops are complemented by other drops that hang downstage from them and

162

provide a three-dimensional effect in the scenery. These usually take the form of cutaway or cutout drops, which go all the way across the stage at the top but which have a portion cut out of the middle so that the actual acting space is open (see Figure 21). In some cases, designers prefer to use a combination of leg and border drops to produce the same effect. A leg is a drop that hangs only to one side of the stage, while the border is a drop that hangs over the top of the scene where a teaser would hang (see Figure 22). The drops are held flat (or nearly so) by weights or pipes inserted into the hem of the drop.

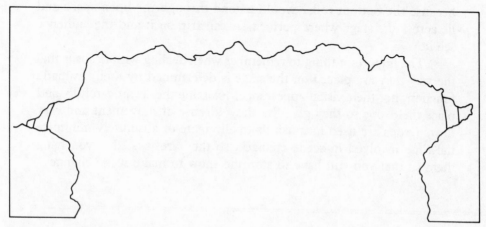

FIGURE 21. Cutaway drop

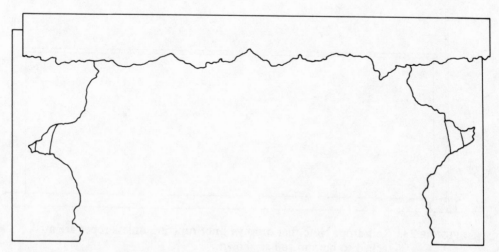

FIGURE 22. Leg and border drops. Used to produce same scene as Figure 21.

To use normal drops, your theatre must have what is called fly space, which is the large open area above the stage itself filled with ropes, pulleys, and pipes. If you have such space, the drops are tied off on the pipes and then lowered or raised out of sight as needed. If you do not, however, and still intend to use drops, you must develop a system for roll drops (see Figure 23), which can be used in very limited overhead fly space. This will not work in all situations; in particular, since the system is self-installed, it requires careful work by the stagehands to keep the drops from tilting or getting wrinkled by irregular rolling. In addition, roll drops cannot be used as cutout drops because the bottom roller would extend through the open space and lie across the stage where performers can trip on it and the audience see it.

The important thing to remember when dealing with drops is that the way they are placed on the stage is determined by their dramatic function, not their visual appearance. Examine the script carefully and place the drops so they give the show a sense of movement and easy flow. Drops are used in musicals to eliminate or absolutely minimize the time involved in scene changes, so they are wasted if you hang them so that you still have to stop the show to make scene changes.

FIGURE 23. Roll drop. Note that drop will not function unless ropes are attached to bottom roll as shown.

LIGHTING

Musicals are probably the hardest kind of theatre to light, because they combine the most difficult parts of the lighting for three completely different kinds of productions—the ballet, the realistic drama, and the variety show—each of which has its own conventions and lighting styles. The combination of ten or more different scenes, each with a different floor space and scenery, almost always using the full width of the stage, with dance scenes, special effects, and star turns, makes outrageous demands on both the lighting designer and the budget.

As a result, musicals demand an enormous amount of equipment. Professional productions use hundreds of lighting instruments: *Hello, Dolly!*, for example, opened in New York with a light plot of about 275 separate instruments, plus a dozen additional trays and groundrows, and used 6 main dimmer boards plus 5 auxiliary circuits for a total of 118 separate dimmer circuits. And that would be regarded as a very simple show in the eighties; *Dreamgirls*, to use a more recent example, used about 950 separate lighting instruments.

Such demands far exceed the capabilities of most organizations and the buildings in which they must perform. Even if the school auditorium (either built by the WPA or, if newer, intended to serve also as gym or cafeteria) should have enough circuits to try such a light plot, no one organization owns enough equipment or can afford to rent it.

Thus, most musicals are forced to adopt a basic simplified lighting system modeled on the one used in professional touring productions. The lighting designer arranges available lights in five steps:

1. Set a *wash*, a simple color and tone of light that covers the entire visible stage in each scene; this gives basic illumination to both the scenery and the acting areas and establishes a simple mood for each scene.

2. Hang the instruments needed for *essential* special effects.

3. Focus down-, back-, and cross-lighting on the most common performing areas—downstage areas, center, and any other commonly used areas in the particular show. This helps give the performers some three-dimensionality and separate them visually from the scenery.

4. Any instruments still unused (usually very few) are divided between

optional special effects and front lighting for the performers in the downstage areas.

5. Because so few instruments remain for front lighting, the lighting designer must add one or more follow-spots, simply so the audience can see the faces of the principals when they speak or sing.

There are a number of dramatic, aesthetic, and even political reasons why the follow-spot should be thought of as a last resort rather than as a fundamental part of musical production (see "Blocking" in Chapter 7). However, there is no denying that it becomes the only practical solution for many problems when groups have limited lighting capabilities.

It is possible to stage a show so that the performers' faces can always be in the available light without follow-spots, even when the lighting instruments are quite limited, but it requires serious effort from both the lighting designer and the stage director. (It also can be done more easily with a unit set rather than with a set of drops because the washes needed to light the drops and full width of the stage in all scenes can be eliminated from the lighting plot, thus freeing up instruments for other uses.) I think it is worth the effort to try for such an ideal, for it establishes a dramatic continuity for the production that regular use of the follow-spots usually destroys. However, it also requires absolutely precise blocking from director and performers, detailed attention to that blocking by the lighting designer (all too rare in any production), and extra rehearsal time on stage during the technical rehearsal period, which many groups simply cannot afford.

SOUND

Except in the smallest of auditoriums with the most sensitive piano accompaniment, most productions will need some sound reinforcement. There are few trained singers in any community, and few musicals that can use trained voices, even if they are available. When professionals depend almost completely on microphones and amplifiers, it is certainly no embarrassment for amateur groups to resort to them as well.

The sound system for a musical should reinforce the natural sound so that everyone in the auditorium can hear clearly. The ideal system is one that no one notices.

Unfortunately, this is very hard to do. The selection and placement of microphones, speakers, and amplifiers differs for every show and every auditorium. There are so many different kinds of equipment available and so many different options to be considered that even a full-time specialist will have problems deciding what will work best in a given situation.

It is also hard to do because of the changing nature of contemporary audiences who have come to believe that all audio problems are solved by making everything louder. This no longer applies exclusively to teenagers who expect to be deafened at music concerts; the people who idolized Elvis are now in their forties, and few from that generation can remember a time when audiences listened to singers or actors who used their natural voices. We were all raised on electric guitars, television and movies played at top volume, and recordings with no volume variation on the radio and stereo. Newer composers are also trained in this way and have come to depend on the sound mixer rather than the performer. Orchestrations are no longer designed to let the sound of the singer come through easily; rather, they are orchestrated like record-studio work—a wall of sound in which the singer's voice is but one sound among many, whose volume is controlled by the audio mixer. Thus, a certain amount of volume is expected by almost everyone no matter how clear the natural sound might be.

In practice, it is impossible to make specific equipment recommendations because of the variety of theatres and shows. However, because most people come to musical production with experience in either nonmusical theatre or concert work, which have little need for sound reinforcement, some basic points may help the beginning group develop a system that will provide practical and genuine sound reinforcement.

A good sound system generally consists of five parts: the microphones, which collect the sound from the performers; the pre-amp (preamplifier), which adjusts the incoming electronic signals to a standard level; the mixer, which allows you to adjust the balance, filtering, and tonal variety among all the microphones; the amplifier, which increases the mixed signal to a level that causes the speaker to reproduce the sound; and the speaker, which converts the electronic signals back into audible sound. Each piece can be connected separately, or the pieces can be found in units that combine several different functions. Most mixers will contain pre-amps, and some will also be part of the larger amplifier. However the pieces may be combined, all five parts of the system are needed for a functioning stage sound system.

The most immediate key to success with this system lies in the microphones. Unless you can collect the sound from the performers to begin with, nothing else will be of any value to the production. Microphones fall into several basic types, some of which are more helpful than others to a musical production.

The most valuable microphone has a cardioid pattern, which means that it picks up sound from an area that is approximately heart-shaped. Thus, it hears sound from one side of the mike, such as the stage, but not from behind it, so that it does not also pick up the sound of the orchestra. It does this better than a typical single-directional microphone, which also hears from only one side, because its pattern is much wider. Where a speaker using a single-directional mike, such as on a speaker's podium, can often disappear simply by turning the head away from the mike, a speaker working with a cardioid of any quality can still be heard several feet on either side of the center of the pattern.

Unfortunately, most schools and auditoriums are usually equipped with less useful microphones such as the omni-directional microphone, which picks up sound approximately equally from all directions. These may be good in some kinds of recording but are valueless in most musical situations because they collect the sound of the orchestra as well as the sound of the singers and thus negate the purpose of the sound system. Music programs often have bi-directional microphones, which pick up sound from two sides. They are thus helpful in recording, but almost worthless in most stage applications.

Professionals recently have made great use of radio microphones, which are worn on the body of the performer, but they do not necessarily solve the problems for the amateur. Such mikes are expensive and complex because they must contain not only a mike, but also a small radio transmitter, batteries to power that transmitter (all of which must be concealed on the performer's body), and a receiver offstage to collect and transfer the signals to the pre-amp and mixer.

This in turn means that you must have several radio microphones; once any one person is individually miked, every other person of any consequence in the cast will expect the same, just as they do with the spotlight. In addition, the need to conceal these mikes inside costumes means that two people cannot share the same mike even if they are never on stage at the same time.

The radio mike also makes problems for the sound operator, who must constantly adjust the sound to balance each of the individual mikes against the sound from the general mikes for the chorus. As radio receivers, they operate on channels with limited range, but which can be interrupted by outside broadcasts. In New York, this has meant that the audience for one show may suddenly hear a singer from the show across the street. In other places (as I have experienced at various times), the interference may come from CB radio operators, police calls, radio baseball games, and television broadcasts. Finally, the microphone goes where the performer goes, and more than one audience has been entertained by fights, cursing, and trips to the bathroom that were broadcast because someone forgot to turn the mike off when the performer left the stage.

A simple, basic system that can provide the starting point for most shows consists of several cardioid microphones placed along the apron of the stage, with narrower single-directional mikes placed to fill in any holes between the patterns. The microphones should be placed as low as possible, only a fraction of an inch off the floor. This often confuses people who want to put the mikes on stands at the level of the singers' mouths, but extensive research and practical experience have shown that mikes placed at this low level collect far more sound than mikes on stands; thus, they provide better sound and do not distract from the visual elements of the performance. There are small foam pads marketed for this purpose on which the microphones may be rested and cushioned, but if you have or can find none of these, any stand will do as long as it is set to place the microphone as near the floor as possible. The mike should never rest directly on the floor, however, as it will then pick up the sound of footsteps and other noise transmitted through the flooring itself.

When choosing amplifiers and speakers, select equipment on which voices sound like voices of people rather than of ghosts or thundering gods in the theatre space. Not all amplifiers and speakers are alike. The great speakers that can produce a throbbing bass line for your rock band may provide mush when asked to work with a musical. Typical public address systems in auditoriums are designed to produce penetrating sound, but with very little quality. This makes the singers' voices loud, but not particularly pleasant to listen to.

Whatever system you use, it should reinforce, not replace, the show. The sound should give the impression of coming from the stage without any delays, so that people in the nearer rows who can hear actual (unmiked) sound from the stage are not distracted by split-second-later repetitions of the sound from the speakers, and people who can hear only the delayed sound from the speakers do not begin to wonder if the performers' voices are dubbed, as in a foreign movie.

Remember, sound reinforcement only reinforces what is already on stage. Don't expect the sound system to solve your performing problems; the singers still must sing the notes and make the tone themselves. *It will make the performance louder, but it will not make it better.*

A passing comment: Clarity projects better than volume. When the words of a song, for example, are not coming through, the solution does not necessarily lie in the volume knob. A different microphone with a better response range, an adjustment of the amplifier for more or less bass, or a speaker with a different response range may solve the problem. In some cases the volume may need to be reduced rather than raised. Many a production has partially deafened audiences (I think especially of productions I have seen of *Grease*) without a single word of the songs being audible. The volume knob is not your only control.

COSTUME

There is no particular style of costuming common to all musicals. Each show has its own practical needs, each show its own visual and artistic style. Even so there are some difficulties most groups face when approaching most musical productions.

The first of these is related to scale. Street clothing is designed to be "read" in daily life at a distance of about five to fifteen feet. Within those distances, the detail of the clothing can be seen, the general impression maintained, and the statement, whatever it might be intended to be, is projected to the other people around you. Stage costume must be read by an audience much farther away, and in musicals, which traditionally use bigger stages and bigger theatres for bigger audiences, the distance at which the costume must project information is often enormous. A gorgeous evening gown that makes its statement perfectly in a nice restaurant may look like a bland blob as a musical costume. Thus, almost all shows must exaggerate and simplify certain aspects of the costume design, so that they can be seen and understood by people in the fifteenth or the fiftieth row.

This is not a requirement of musicals *per se*; it is simply a fact of life when dealing with large spaces. If your show is in a large theatre, the costume problems are different than they would be for the same show in a small one. Costumes that work perfectly for *Camelot* in a 1500-seat house may be too simple or too exaggerated for the same show in a 500-seat house.

A second problem area more consistently associated with musicals is the fact that many of the costumes must be worn while dancing. For the most part, even in the active eighties, normal tailoring of clothing does not allow the wearer the free movement needed for dancing or some other on-stage activities. In musicals, fashion styles must be adjusted to allow for the possibility of dance, and the less experienced the dancers, the more the costume must be modified.

The choreographer must accept some limitations from the costumes. Anna in *The King and I* wears the rigid, corseted, hoop-skirted dresses of her time, and her personality is reflected in those firm, upright, corseted clothes. That's why her big dance number is a polka; it's a dance that can be done in an upright position. No choreographer who vaguely understands the show would try to force her into dips and swirls or leaps or Bob Fosse-styled contortions. But in many other cases the costume design must be modified so that the dancers can work, rather than vice versa.

This makes rentals a particular problem. Of all the terrors that face a cast during tech rehearsals, none is so great as the moment when they put on the costumes and discover that they can't do some of the dance movements in them. If these are rental costumes, they can't be significantly modified; this in turn means that two or three days before the show opens, the dancers have to rechoreograph and relearn a number to replace something it took them six to eight *weeks* to learn. Thus, if it is at all practical, it is often to your advantage to make your own dance costumes, even if you rent all the rest of the costumes for the show.

Most musicals require each character to wear several different costumes. This means there must be someplace where the actors can change costumes during the show. In some cases, these changes cannot be done in dressing rooms because there isn't time for the performer to get to the dressing room, change, and still get back for the next entrance. Such quick changes require two important aids. First, you must have dressers waiting to help the performer(s) make those changes; how many dressers are required depends on the number of quick changes that must be made at any given time. Second, you must be able to guarantee a certain amount of privacy. How much privacy is required will depend on the personality, age, and experience of the performers, but some is always required. Plan such things as carefully as possible to keep quick changes to a minimum.

The most important part of the costume, and the part of the costume most often overlooked, is the shoe. Everyone in a musical moves, with most people either dancing or at least giving the impression of dancing. The kind of movement possible is limited by the shoes worn. As a result, shoes must be considered and planned for at every stage in the rehearsal. This is essential in all groups, but most important in schools, where many of the performers have worn nothing but tennis shoes or sandals for the past ten years of their lives and have no idea how to stand, much less move around, in anything else. And there are very few musicals written for casts in tennis shoes. Shoes from periods that are bulky and heavy must be modified for movement. When they cannot be modified to any significant degree, all movement must be adjusted so that it can be accomplished with the available footwear. The cast should rehearse in these shoes, if possible, from day one of rehearsals. This is particularly important for school-age casts or casts that must wear unusual footwear, such as the period boots for *Two Gentlemen of Verona* or the sandals of the Siamese in *The King and I*.

Finally, remember that all costumes get dirty, but musical costumes get dirtiest. Dancers sweat, and singers usually sweat even more from sheer nervous tension. Any costume that comes in contact with the skin must be cleanable if you expect to survive tech rehearsals, dress rehearsals, and a run of even a few nights. In most cases this means washable; dry cleaning is far too expensive for most show budgets. Fortunately, there are an enormous number of washable modern fabrics that can be used in the costumes. If a certain look demands nonwashable materials, be sure to include a separate interior layer of costume that can be removed and washed regularly. For rented costumes, be sure that the performers wear underwear that can soak up the sweat, and use dress shields wherever possible unless you are absolutely sure you can wash them. In most cases you will receive costumes with no cleaning labels, in which case assume they are not washable.

MAKEUP

Many people worry about learning how to do Musical Comedy Makeup. There is no such thing. The two functions of makeup are to compensate for the lighting by restoring natural color to skin that the lighting would wash out, and to define and project some element of characterization that helps to visually define the person portrayed. In any show, the type of makeup used will depend on a number of different factors such as the style of the show itself, the size of the auditorium, the nature and color of the lighting used for the production, and the relative age and appearance of each individual performer. Shows in schools tend to need more makeup than shows in community theatres, because community groups often have people of the proper age for most of the roles. Musicals often require a certain amount of exaggeration, but this is due to the size of the auditorium or the style of the individual show, not to the fact that the show is a musical.

The practical problems associated with musical makeup are usually results of the size and relative inexperience of the cast. The problem is to get makeup on forty or fifty people, most of whom have never used stage makeup or learned its basic principles. Most groups resort to the use of a makeup crew, a group of people who line up the members of the cast and put the makeup on for them. This is practical because it is fast, if the makeup crew does in fact know what it is doing (which is not always the case in practice), but it is not necessarily ideal.

Especially in schools, each person should put on his or her own makeup. Boys dislike this, as a general rule, primarily because they think it makes them look like a sissy of some kind. I have found that they prefer crews simply because they enjoy having all those girls leaning over them and devoting all their attention to their needs. However, once it is clear that *everyone* is expected to do his or her own makeup, the boys quickly accept that. This still demands time to teach everyone how to do the makeup needed, but again I have found that it takes little more time than it takes to teach a makeup crew to do the same work, and it gives a number of advantages. Not the least of these is that some of the people in the cast will be in the next cast and will thus know how to deal with their own makeup in all succeeding productions. In addition, a performer who puts on his or her own makeup starts to think about the character and the performance, while a performer who has someone else apply the makeup invariably spends the makeup session in socializing. You get better performances when people think about the show before each performance than you do when they spend the time before the curtain talking about their private lives or the state of the nation.

Remember that the only real test of the makeup is the eye. Whatever the books say (or classes, or the other shows you may have seen), you must make the makeup work under your lighting in your auditorium. When you are designing and the cast is learning the makeup, always go out on the stage to check it under the lights that will be used in performance. Ideally, a good makeup projects the desired information to the last seat in the house without looking like a mask to the first seat. In a large auditorium this is difficult, and if you use a follow-spot, with its harsh light, it is practically impossible. However, you can design for the middle of the house. If the performer still looks like he or she is wearing artificial makeup (except in stylized shows like *Godspell*) from the middle of the house, the makeup is too strong; if you can't detect any features in the face from the same seat, the makeup is too weak.

One other point: One of the most persistent complaints from costumers is the way the people who rent the costumes use makeup. Most makeup is extremely difficult to remove from clothing, especially when it has been caked on for several days. Makeup should be applied to all exposed areas of the skin, not just to the face, so that all the skin seems to belong to the same person. But there is no reason it should also be applied to the costumes. Be sure the cast puts on makeup before putting on their complete costume, to avoid dribbling makeup all over the costume. Be even more careful to see that there are washable layers between the makeup and the costume wherever possible—shirts with collars under jackets, slips and chemises inside blouses, and so on.

STORAGE

The most wonderful scenery and props in the world are worthless if you can't get them on and off the stage when you need them. Because musicals usually involve a number of scenery pieces, the storage space needed for them when they are not on stage must be an important factor in their design and construction.

Drops of course go into the fly space, and as long as the fly space is high enough for your drops, they present no storage problems. This is one of the reasons they are so common in musical productions. But wagons, furniture, and individual pieces of scenery must fit some-place backstage. Unfortunately, so must the performers. Unless you plan so that there is a specific place for each piece of scenery and each prop and still leave entrance and exit space for the performers, the show will come to a screeching halt every time any change must be made.

In addition, each specific backstage storage position must allow enough room for all the other scenery and props to be moved about freely. For example, in *My Fair Lady*, Higgins's study appears five different times. Normally the study is composed of a drop plus props and furniture on wagons or carried on individually. This stays on stage after its first appearance, behind the drop for the scene-in-one for Doolittle's song. But after its second scene, at least part of it must be cleared for the Ascot scenes. When these wagons or pieces of furniture go offstage, they cannot go in front of the pieces needed for the Ascot set, because they would block that set from coming on. At the same time, they cannot go into the space vacated by the Ascot set either, because they would now be blocked from going back on stage for their next appearance. Such things must be planned meticulously by the designer and the stage manager, or the entire production will collapse in performance.

PRODUCTION BOOK

Each production should have a complete production book. This is the Bible of the show, and it is the responsibility of the stage manager to prepare, maintain, and then use it properly.

A complete production book includes the following:

1. The complete libretto of the show
2. Notations of all blocking
3. Notations of all significant business added
4. Indications of all light and sound effects cues
5. Indications of all cues to be given to any offstage personnel, such as warnings to performers of upcoming scenes or warnings to stage crews for scene changes
6. Directions for all scene changes, in detail, including not only who makes changes and when, but also a complete description of the finished stage picture
7. Production schedule, all rehearsal schedules, and any crew schedules used in the production

The production book is used by the stage manager to run the show. It should allow him or her, in effect, to guarantee that the show seen on any given night is the same as on any other night (as near as is humanly possible). If there are disputes after rehearsals are finished as to the way any part of the show is intended to run, the production book is the final authority. It should be so complete that in theory an assistant or even a complete stranger could take over the stage manager's job in an emergency and still know everything necessary to get the show on and running properly (see Figure 24).

The rule for any production book is: When in doubt, write it down. Each stage manager will have a slightly different method of notation and abbreviation. Sometimes things can be noted in words, sometimes in drawings. But everything that needs to be repeated in a consistent manner should be noted somewhere for reference in case of problems, emergencies, disagreements, or forgetfulness. Leave nothing to memory.

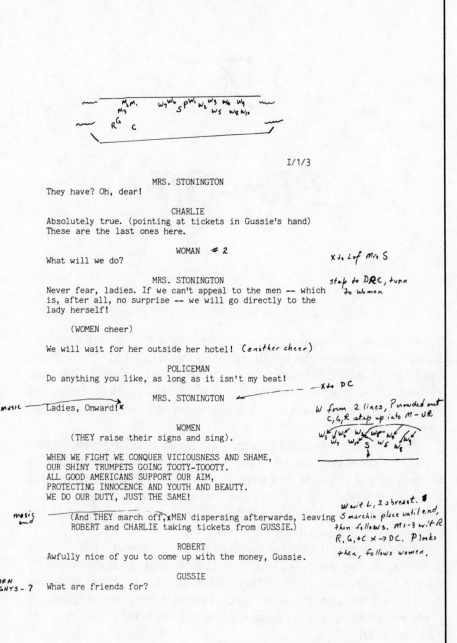

I/1/3

MRS. STONINGTON
They have? Oh, dear!

CHARLIE
Absolutely true. (pointing at tickets in Gussie's hand)
These are the last ones here.

WOMAN #2
What will we do?   *X to L of Mrs S*

MRS. STONINGTON   *step to DRC, turn*
Never fear, ladies. If we can't appeal to the men -- which   *to women*
is, after all, no surprise -- we will go directly to the
lady herself!

    (WOMEN cheer)

We will wait for her outside her hotel! *(another cheer)*

POLICEMAN
Do anything you like, as long as it isn't my beat!
                                                    — X to DC

music — MRS. STONINGTON *←*
Ladies, Onward!*x*   *W form 2 lines, P crowded out*
                                            C, G, R step up into M - UR

WOMEN
    (THEY raise their signs and sing).

WHEN WE FIGHT WE CONQUER VICIOUSNESS AND SHAME,
OUR SHINY TRUMPETS GOING TOOTY-TOOOTY.
ALL GOOD AMERICANS SUPPORT OUR AIM,
PROTECTING INNOCENCE AND YOUTH AND BEAUTY.
WE DO OUR DUTY, JUST THE SAME!

music   W exit L, 2 abreast.
end   (And THEY march off,*x*MEN dispersing afterwards, leaving *S march in place until end,*
         ROBERT and CHARLIE taking tickets from GUSSIE.) *then follows. M1-3 with R*
                                            R, G, +C X → DC. P looks
ROBERT   *then, follows women.*
Awfully nice of you to come up with the money, Gussie.

GUSSIE
WARN
LIGHTS - 7 What are friends for?

9

Play-Off

If you followed the production process suggested in the previous chapters, the gleam in the eye that got you started should still be there. The production will have been an enormous amount of work, but even so, most of the people involved will think it was worth it. In fact, if you listen at the cast party, you'll hear more than one voice asking, "What'll we do next year?"

Most amateur musical productions begin as a single-shot idea: Let's do a show and see what happens. While the production is in process, no one has time or energy to think about doing it again. But if that first production is successful, many people will immediately start looking for ways to institutionalize the process—to arrange for similar productions on a regular basis.

In most cases, the people involved in a musical will work through an existing organization—a school, a church, a community theatre, a charity organization. Some of these, such as schools and community theatres, will already have some kind of theatrical organization system in place. For these groups what follows may be helpful, but it is not really essential.

At some point, however, many people may find a need to establish their own organization devoted primarily or completely to the production of future musicals. For these, the following points should be considered.

THE PRODUCING ORGANIZATION

Any organization that produces theatrical productions, musical or nonmusical, must be organized to deal with two different time scales. One of these has to do with the individual production while the other has to deal with several different productions over the life of the organization. The organization must also perform in two places at the same time—on stage and within some community. That community may consist of a particular school, church, group of associates, or the town as a whole, but as we have seen, the community is an important factor in every production.

Thus, the musical production group needs two different and overlapping organizations: a production organization, which consists of the staff and cast members who actually plan, rehearse, and perform each musical seen on stage, but who change for each individual production; and an administrative organization that deals with the production in the context of the community and serves through several different productions. We have examined in detail what the production organization does in previous chapters.

Administrative Staff

The administrative staff of an organization serves two essential functions that can be served in no other way.

1. It provides an organizational framework that makes the musical production the work of a group rather than merely of a few individuals; this makes it easier to attract new people to auditions and for staff positions while at the same time guaranteeing that there will always be a few experienced people available as each production begins.
2. When properly incorporated as a nonprofit organization under local state laws, it serves as a legal entity separate from any individuals in the production; this relieves the individuals of legal liability in case of financial or legal difficulties.

The administrative organization of each group will be slightly different, depending on the legal requirements for incorporation and the needs of the local organization itself. However, a minimal, efficient administrative staff for a musical producing group would include the following:

1. Financial Officer—normally called a treasurer or business manager. This is the person who ultimately signs all the checks and keeps all the financial records, who counts and watches the money.
2. Executive Officer—normally called a chairman or a president. This is the person who speaks for the organization as a whole. Generally, this person provides the legal signature for contracts entered into by the organization. In most cases, this executive officer will not be directly involved in the actual production of the show. In schools, for example, this will be the principal, while in church-related groups it may be the minister or the head of the board of lay officers that administers the church's temporal activities. In community theatre groups, this executive officer may or may not be an actor or other production participant; most groups find it helpful if the executive officer is more concerned with being a public spokesman and fundraiser than with being on stage.
3. Advisory or Supervisory Board—usually called a board of directors. This group makes decisions that affect the organization as a whole and represents the members of the group, as opposed to only the staff of one particular show, in some way. It will determine budgets and financial arrangements, approve contracts, hire staff where such staff is needed, and usually at least approve if not select the shows to be produced.

Most groups eventually include additional officers: a secretary to keep records and deal with correspondence, a vice-president to act when the primary executive officer is unavailable, a legal advisor to deal with all contracts and licenses, and the like. However, an administrative group can function in the early stages of organization with only the two officers and a small board of directors.

This administrative organization may be elected, appointed, accepted as volunteers, or formed in any combination of these three methods. Some of the people may be involved in a particular production, although most will not and should not be.

In a good administrative staff each person will have a particular area of expertise, with one person specializing in financial accounting, another in fundraising, another in technical planning or supervision of facilities, another in publicity, and so on. Their function is to plan and advise for the organization as a whole and to consider all problems and solutions in terms of the traditions and the future of the organization rather than in terms of any individual production.

When dealing with individual productions, actual procedures may be very flexible. In some cases, the administrative staff will tend to leave as much of the operation of the organization as possible in the hands of the production staff. In others, they will try to take part in almost every decision. Most boards fall somewhere between, and each board must feel its own way in a particular situation. Several of the works listed in the Bibliography will provide detailed and helpful information about the daily operation of a theatre administration. But however administrative boards operate, it is important to remember that they are essential; someone must provide a vision that goes beyond opening night. If you intend to produce a series of musicals, rather than only one musical, then the formation and development of a good administrative organization is essential.

At the same time, it is important to recognize that certain predictable conflicts among the various staff members may arise in even the best situations. Most of these have been discussed in detail in the previous chapters and need not be repeated here. However, it might be helpful to remember a very important general principle.

Musicals are exciting to produce precisely because they offer so many different opportunities to use so many different skills and talents. The most persistent organizational problems arise when members of the administrative staff forget this.

The most common complaints heard about theatre administrations are not about money, although that would seem to be the most likely level of conflict; rather, members of both the production staffs and the casts of individual shows complain most often about what they consider interference in their areas of expertise.

Everyone who has worked in amateur theatre has a horror story to tell, so I need not list my own here. Far too many organizations operate on the unspoken assumption that anyone willing to work for them must be constantly monitored, supervised, and guarded against at all times. Naturally enough, they have regular problems keeping good production staff. The most important way to find and keep good production staff members is to respect their decisions and let them do the jobs for which they were selected.

There are limits on what the various staff members can do, most of which are budgetary and have been explained in detail in previous chapters. Some organizations have additional limits as a result of the nature of the organization itself—dancers in school or church group productions cannot be asked to go topless or to mime sexual intercourse, for example. It is well within the province of the administrative staff's role to hold the production staff to those limitations. Within those limits, however, the staff must be trusted. If you have no intentions of letting the designers design or the directors direct, then do the jobs yourselves; don't waste time, money, and energy finding someone else to do them. People who feel creative and fulfilled will do good work and want to come back again; those who don't will not return again when needed in the future and often may not even finish the production itself. As long as they stay within the budget and the officially stated policy of the organization, let them do the job for which they were selected in whatever seems to them to be the best manner.

Licensing Agencies for Musicals

Scripts and librettos for most famous, Broadway-style musicals are available through one of four agencies:

> Tams-Witmark Music Library, Inc.
> 560 Lexington Ave.
> New York, NY 10022

Tams handles most of the widely known "golden-age" musicals and specializes in big Broadway hits. As a result, it has in the recent past developed a reputation as hard to deal with. I have found them to be sticklers for contract rules, but no more unresponsive than any other organization in my own dealings. They also rent only "sides" (see Chapter 3), which makes their rehearsal materials very awkward, but if you want a familiar show, this is where to start looking.

> Music Theatre International
> 1350 Avenue of the Americas
> New York, NY 10019

Somewhat less aggressive in its marketing and generally more responsive to individual problems, MTI also deals in Broadway hits for the most part, with the most attractive part of its library built around shows by Sondheim, Loesser, and Willson. It has also taken on many of the newer revue-type shows and most of the early off-Broadway, small-group hits.

> Rodgers & Hammerstein Theatre Library
> 598 Madison Ave.
> New York, NY 10022

R&H deals in exactly that—shows written by Rodgers, Hammerstein, or Rodgers and Hammerstein.

Samuel French, Inc.
25 West 45th St.
New York, NY 10036

One of the oldest play agencies in the country, Samuel French has been comparatively slow in developing its musical catalog. With a few exceptions, it has tended to specialize in shows that were not quite hits, or were off-Broadway hits, with a number of less well-known shows tailored for schools and community groups with limited resources.

Less famous musicals, but often of good quality, can also be found from the following sources:

Dramatic Publishing Co.
311 Washington St.
Woodstock, IL 60098

Long a major agency in the school market, DPC has recently moved aggressively into adult-oriented works to complement its popular, large line of plays and musicals written for schools and children's groups. Thus, schools will usually find some good musicals tailored for typical production problems they face, and adult groups may find some interesting Broadway and London material as well. Extremely efficient and eager to help.

Broadway Play Publishing, Inc.
249 West 29th St.
New York, NY 10001

A brand-new company, still with a very limited catalog, with some musicals from regional theatre and English sources.

Theatre Maximus
1650 Broadway
New York, NY 10019

A very small company whose primary business seems to be the licensing of *Godspell*, although it does handle some other material as well.

Anchorage Press
PO Box 8067
New Orleans, LA 70181

Baker's Plays
100 Chauncy St.
Boston, MA 02111

Centerstage Press
4638 E. Shea Blvd.
Suite B-150
Phoenix, AZ 85028

Contemporary Drama Service
Box 457
1529 Brook Drive
Downers Grove, IL 60515

I.E. Clark
Box 246
Schulenburg, TX 78956

Performance Publishing Co.
978 McLean Blvd.
Elgin, IL 60120
(Recently purchased by Baker's Plays, its catalog may soon be combined with Baker's)

Pioneer Drama Service
PO Box 22555
Denver, CO 80222

These agencies all deal primarily with plays for schools, children, or groups with limited resources. The musicals they offer vary in quality, but then so do the more famous Broadway shows. Almost all of the shows they offer will be comparatively simple to stage and suitable for young or "family" audiences.

Selected
Bibliography

Books

Anderson, Barbara and Cletus. *Costume Design*. New York: Holt, Rinehart and Winston, 1984. An attractive, extensive, and well-illustrated introduction to both the theory and practice of modern costume-design techniques.

Balk, H. Wesley. *The Complete Actor-Singer: Training for Music Theater*. Minneapolis: University of Minnesota Press, 2nd ed. 1985. Aimed at opera students, it offers considerable help and useful advice for the musical comedy cast member who is comfortable with singing but terrified about acting and moving.

Bay, Howard. *Scene Design*. New York: Drama Book Specialists (Publishers), 1978. A major Broadway designer discusses both his career and the theory and practice of design in one of the very few books to devote significant attention to the unique aspects of scenery and lighting design for musicals.

Burris-Meyer, Harold, and Edward C. Cole. *Scenery for the Theatre*, 2d rev. ed. Boston: Little, Brown & Co., 1972. The ultimate scenery text, especially complete and detailed.

Collison, David. *Stage Sound*, 2d rev. ed. New York: Drama Books, 1982. Still somewhat British in its orientations and discussions of specific equipment, but the only serious text in the field, quite clear and helpful.

Corson, Richard. *Stage Makeup*, 6th ed. Englewood Cliffs, N.J.: Prentice-Hall, 1981. Practically everything you need to know about almost any possible aspect of stage makeup.

Craig, David. *On Singing Onstage*. New York: Schirmer Books, 1978. For the actor who is afraid to sing, with excellent advice on analyzing, dramatizing, and performing songs in theatrical productions.

Dean, Alexander, and Lawrence Carra. *Fundamentals of Play Directing*, 4th ed. New York: Holt, Rinehart and Winston, 1980. Although in many ways I prefer earlier editions, this still remains one of the most practical stage-directing books, especially strong in blocking and focusing techniques for the proscenium stage, where most musicals must be performed.

Dryden, Deborah. *Fabric Painting and Dyeing for the Theatre*. New York: Drama Book Specialists (Publishers), 1981. A compendium of techniques that are often extremely helpful to the designer trying to cope with the large scale and colorful world of most musical productions.

Engel, Lehman. *Getting the Show On*. New York: Schirmer Books, 1983. A reissue of an earlier edition, short on practical advice but with a valuable long descriptive summary of practically every Broadway musical available from the forties through the late sixties.

Gillette, A. S. and J. Michael. *Stage Scenery: Its Construction and Rigging*, 3rd ed. New York: Harper & Row, 1981. Especially helpful for people trying to cope with drops and fly lofts for a complex musical production.

Grote, David. *Script Analysis*. Belmont, Cal.: Wadsworth, 1984. A detailed and practical method for understanding the dramatic script and extracting the maximum amount of information from it before you begin rehearsals.

Gruver, Bert. *The Stage Manager's Handbook*, revised by Frank Hamilton. New York: Drama Book Specialists (Publishers), 1972. Written for the professional, but with much detailed and helpful advice that also applies to the complex and critical role of stage manager of an amateur production.

Hodge, Francis. *Play Directing: Analysis, Communication, and Style*. Englewood Cliffs, N.J.: Prentice-Hall, 1971. An extremely intelligent, detailed discussion of the director's job, especially valuable on style and the director's relations with actors and other staff.

Hoggett, Chris. *Stage Crafts*. New York: St. Martin's Press, 1975. A meticulously illustrated and surprisingly complete little book, especially helpful to people or groups with little practical production experience of any kind. It uses metric examples, but the drawings are extremely clear and more than compensate.

Humphrey, Doris. *The Art of Making Dances*. New York: Grove Press, 1978. Written by one of the most famous choreographers of modern dance, this remains one of the most stimulating and helpful introductions to the planning of dramatic dance of any kind as well as to the use of stage space and movement of any kind within that space; recommended for both choreographers and directors.

Ingham, Rosemary and Elizabeth Covey. *The Costumer's Handbook: How to Make All Kinds of Costumes*. Englewood Cliffs, N.J.: Prentice-Hall, 1980. Very practical aid in costume organization and construction, including helpful lists of sources and suppliers across the country for theatrical fabrics, wigs, shoes, and specialty items.

Kenton, Warren. *Stage Properties and How to Make Them*, rev. ed. New York: Drama Book Specialists (Publishers), 1978. Good practical advice on simple, effective, and generally cheap ways to make props that are often difficult to find or too expensive to purchase or rent, with lots of illustrations.

Kosarin, Oscar. *The Singing Actor: How to Be a Success in Musical Theater and Nightclubs*. Englewood Cliffs, N.J.: Prentice-Hall, 1983. Although it might more clearly be called *The Acting Singer*, a generally helpful book of advice for making dramatic sense of the song, both in a show and when singing in other contexts, simpler and more direct than Balk.

Miller, James H. *Stage Lighting in the Boondocks*. Downer's Grove, Ill.: Arthur Meriwether, Inc., 1981. In spite of some reservations about some of the advice, this remains the only lighting book that mentions the fact that most organizations neither operate in state-of-the-art facilities nor have budgets for extensive equipment rentals, and it can be very helpful to groups with rotten facilities or who must produce in halls, churches, and other spaces not intended for stage work.

Newman, Danny. *Subscribe Now!* New York: Theatre Communications Group, 1977. A guide originally written for professional nonprofit theatres to use in fundraising and ticket sales campaigns, it has excellent advice in these areas for any performing group.

Parker, W. Oren and Harvey K. Smith. *Scene Design and Stage Lighting*, 4th ed. New York: Holt, Rinehart & Winston, 1979. One of the most widely used basic texts in theatrical stagecraft techniques.

Pektal, Lynn. *Designing and Painting for the Theatre*. New York: Holt, Rinehart and Winston, 1975. Not so much on design as on painting, but the painting techniques, especially for drops, are detailed and well illustrated.

Rosenthal, Jean and Lael Wertenbaker. *The Magic of Light*. Boston: Little, Brown & Co., 1972. Excellent introduction to most lighting techniques, illustrated through a good set of photos, includes detailed copies and explanations of New York production light plots.

Sellman, Hunton D. and Merill J. Lessley. *Essentials of Stage Lighting*, 2d ed. Englewood Cliffs, N.J.: Prentice-Hall, 1982. Detailed discussion of lighting techniques and equipment.

Stern, Lawrence. *School and Community Theater Management: A Handbook for Survival*, new ed. Boston: Allyn and Bacon, 1979. A help for keeping the organization working so that shows can get into production.

Tompkins, Julia. *Stage Costumes and How to Make Them*. Boston: Plays, Inc., 1976. The best "simple" method of costume pattern making and construction available; extremely helpful to relatively inexperienced costumers and to groups with limited budgets.

Welker, David. *Stagecraft: A Handbook for Organization, Construction, and Manage-

ment. Boston: Allyn and Bacon, 1977. Exactly what the title says; especially strong in methods of organizing and operating the scene shop and backstage areas.

Wilfred, Thomas. *Projected Scenery: A Technical Manual*. New York: Drama Book Specialists (Publishers), 1965. In desperate need of updating, but the only detailed introduction to an imaginative method that can be used in many theatres to simplify or eliminate drops.

Magazines, journals, organizational newsletters, and occasional publications

Dramatics, published by International Thespian Society, 3368 Central Parkway, Cincinnati, OH 45225. A general-interest theatre magazine written for high school theatre students and teachers, but of some interest to others in the field as well. Students receive the magazine as part of Thespian membership, but subscriptions are available to nonmembers.

Theatre Crafts, 33 East Minor St., Emmaus, PA 18049. A well-written and illustrated general theatrical production magazine reporting on scenery, lighting, and costume developments in both professional and educational theatres.

Theatre Crafts Directory, A regularly revised publication from *Theatre Crafts* magazine that provides updated lists of suppliers of stage materials and instruments for sale or rental from across the nation.

Theatre Design and Technology, published by the U.S. Institute for Theatre Technology, 330 W. 42nd St., New York, NY 10036. Covers much the same general areas as *Theatre Crafts* but from a somewhat more specialized and technical viewpoint. Membership required.

In addition, the American Community Theatre Association and Secondary School Theatre Association, both divisions of the American Theatre Association, 1010 Wisconsin Ave. NW, Suite 630, Washington, DC 20007, both publish newsletters and/or journals dealing with problems and interests of their members, which often deal with musicals and related productions. Membership required for personal subscriptions.

TYPICAL MUSICALS FOR AMATEUR GROUPS

The shows most often performed by amateurs are the same as those performed by professionals, with about a five-to-twenty-year delay. In general, when school or community theatre groups decide to do a musical, they will pick one of about four dozen well-known shows, almost all of which originated in New York, simply because "Broadway" and "musical" are all but inseparable in the public mind.

Although the selection process is detailed and complex, as described in Chapter 2, the following list of these popular musicals may be helpful to many beginners. The list includes the most generally performed shows and a brief description of pertinent information about each. The information includes the following categories:

1. Agent—the company from whom copies can be obtained and with whom royalty and rental agreements must be negotiated. (Addresses for these are listed on page 183.)

2. Type—basic emphasis of the musical production (discussed below).

3. Period—the period and place in which the show is costumed, to suggest potential costuming costs.

4. Set—scenery convention around which the show is organized, that is, drop, unit, or single unchanging set (see Chapter 3). Note that this does not mean you must use only that one kind of scenery—a full set of drops for a drop show, for example. Variations, simplifications, and modifications are possible with practically every show.

5. Size—cast size stated approximately, because many shows have roles that may be doubled or have very flexible choral requirements.

6. Attractions—the parts of the show that audience or production groups, or both, seem to find most valuable or effective.

7. Problems—the parts of the show with which most amateur groups are likely to have difficulties.

It should be stressed that this is not a recommended list of shows. It is simply a brief introduction to those shows that are most likely to occur to people looking for a musical to do. As indicated on page 185, there are an enormous number of musicals available for amateur production, many of which are designed specifically for those with limited space, budgets, or experience, or for specialized audiences. This includes shows with a single simple set, inexpensive costume demands, music in limited singing ranges that put no strain on untrained singers, accompaniment arranged for piano only, and/or librettos without any mention of sex or four-letter words or of interest to small children, high school students, or specific minorities. Such shows may fit your needs far better than any of the shows described; only their unfamiliarity excludes them from this brief introductory list. In similar fashion, a number of Broadway musicals I much admire and which I think could be well done by many groups are not listed either. The list has to end somewhere, so it considers only the obvious titles.

BASIC TYPES OF SHOWS

Although we think of musicals as a single, uniform kind of theatre, there are in fact at least six different types. Each of these has its own attractions and its own production problems, and it may help the beginner starting the selection process to understand them.

Most of these six types overlap in some way, with only a few shows obviously limited to a single type. Most star vehicles, for example, at least go through the motions of being a book show, and many book shows will require important elements of spectacle and/or star roles. The categories below simply indicate the primary emphasis of the production. It is important for any group considering any show to understand this emphasis, so that the strengths of the organization can be used to best advantage in the production and the weaknesses minimized.

1. The Book Show

For many people the only *real* musical is the book musical. It is to these that we turn when we talk of a golden age in American musicals, when a revolution in audience tastes led by Rodgers and Hammerstein and Lerner and Loewe gave us shows that tried to fully integrate music, drama, dance, and spectacle in a single, whole dramatic work.

Although these works have elements of spectacle and often began with stars in major roles, they are organized around their stories. Audiences can respond to the plot of the show as well as to the production itself. Many of these shows are not even comedies in the usual sense of the term, using very serious story lines like *West Side Story*'s use of *Romeo and Juliet*, *Cabaret*'s bitter portrait of pre-Hitler Germany, or *Sweeney Todd*'s revival of the horrors of earnest melodrama. Others maintain their roots in comedy, but demand real characterizations and the appearance of reality in many of their nonmusical moments.

Consequently, book shows tend to require performers who can act as well as sing and dance, and often will require such talents in the majority of the cast. Where a star vehicle will share musical numbers among a very few performers, a book show like *West Side Story* passes them around among nine solo-caliber singer/dancer/actors in addition to a large, extremely talented chorus who also play distinct minor characters.

2. The Spectacle Show

Since *The Black Crook* laid the foundations of American musical theatre, we have passed through periods when productions were dominated by gorgeous scenery, flashy costumes, spectacular dance numbers, and often large numbers of women in skimpy costumes. The first wave came in the late nineteenth century, the second in the twenties and thirties when Ziegfeld, Carroll, and other producers gave us follies, scandals, and other forgettable shows with unforgettable songs by Gershwin, Rodgers and Hart, Porter, Berlin, and Kern among others. These faded for a time with the book musicals stimulated by *Oklahoma!*, but are making a new comeback in the late seventies and eighties with such generally plotless successes as *Jesus Christ Superstar, Evita, Dancin'*, and *Cats*, and such lightly plotted, spectacle-heavy shows as *Forty-Second Street*.

In this type of musical, the show is the show; no one pays much attention to the dramatic aspects, if such aspects even exist. What counts are the scenery, the costumes, the dance numbers each more spectacular than the last, and whatever gimmicks or special effects can be added. The book is there merely as a framework for holding all the pieces together and because contemporary audiences are thought to demand a book of some kind.

These generally provide greater problems for most amateur groups than any other type because they strike where the group is weakest—money, technical skill, and facilities. Without the spectacle, the show doesn't really exist any more, no matter what other attractions may exist in the script, and most groups are unable to afford the spectacle.

3. The Star Vehicle

Some shows have stars in them, others make stars of relative unknowns who rise to prominence in them, but some shows are made by and for their stars. The dialogue, the musical numbers, and the characterizations of almost all the characters, not just the lead role, are controlled and shaped by a star to fit the talents of that particular performer and to show that talent in the best possible light at all times. Some star vehicles outlast their initial stars (*Gypsy*) while others close quickly in professional productions when the star is no longer available (*Coco, Wildcat*).

These shows may have other strengths, but at the core of the show is *one* stellar performance. *Annie Get Your Gun* and *Gypsy*, for example, are carefully tailored to the unusual and very specific talents of Ethel Merman, as *Funny Girl* is designed to show off Barbra Streisand. The essential key is that one person appears in the majority of all musical numbers—Tevye in *Fiddler on the Roof*, for example, is in nine of the twelve numbers, Rose in *Gypsy* is in eight of thirteen. (By contrast, in *My Fair Lady*, a book show with stars, Eliza and Higgins each sing only five of the fourteen separate songs and share one other.) This emphasis on a single person makes two problems for any amateur group.

Many local people may be as talented as the original stars, but that talent will always be different from that of the original star. This means that some parts of the show will simply never quite work in the expected way. Also, many cast members and people in the organization come to resent the expenditure of so much effort and money for the primary benefit of a single person.

4. The Ensemble Show

In general, an ensemble show will be a book show but with a difference: It will almost completely forego spectacle, and most of the non-chorus roles will be about the same size and difficulty. Very often, there will not be a chorus distinct from the principals. These are usually low-budget shows following in the tradition of *The Fantasticks*, which is the modern progenitor of the genre, and *Godspell*, perhaps at present the most popular of such works. In recent years, larger budgets have made larger Broadway-level successes of such shows, as with *A Chorus Line, Hair,* and *Company* while some others like *The Robber Bridegroom* grow out of the regional theatre milieu.

The comparatively small casts, unit sets, and resulting comparatively small budgets make these shows especially attractive to amateur groups. However, they also tend to need a comparatively large group of equally talented, equally egoed performers, lots of imagination in staging, and much more intensive and thoughtful publicity campaigns to draw audiences than the more familiar book musicals or star vehicles.

5. The Revue

The revue is a musical without a plot. In Ziegfeld's days the revue was a spectacle show, but in recent years it has changed enormously. The old revues were essentially vaudeville shows, alternating music, comedy routines, and production numbers. Newer revues such as *Cole, Side by Side by Sondheim, Sophisticated Ladies,* or *Jacques Brel Is Alive and Well and Living in Paris,* tend to concentrate almost completely on music, usually by a single composer. Others concentrate on a single theme with music by several composers, as in *Working,* or a single composer, as in *Runaways* or *You're a Good Man, Charlie Brown.*

The primary attraction of these is the music, which tends to be familiar, even nostalgic. They require mainly singers, which makes them very attractive for beginning groups. But they also tend to work best in very small theatres, where their lack of dramatic interest or spectacle is compensated for by the intimacy of the performance. They also tend not to draw large audiences, because they are both less well-known to the broad general audience and have smaller casts than the classic book musicals.

6. *The Operetta*

The operetta is an oddity to modern audiences and hard to define. It has a book, but in contemporary terms usually a rather silly one. It sometimes shares the musical's structural conventions (see Chapter 3), and at other times simply drops music in, apparently at random. The one genuine constant is that it demands trained singers. Perhaps the best way to define it is that its principals are almost always sopranos and tenors with two-octave ranges, while other musicals tend to be written for mezzos and baritones with about an octave in range.

In the operetta, color and spectacle are important because the locale is usually exotic, such as Morocco in *Desert Song* or Japan in *The Mikado*. Compared to book musicals, however, there tend to be few scenery and costume changes. The real spectacle is the singing. Many of the songs are designed not for character exposition but for exposing the performer's ability. There is also a very clear division of roles: principals sing and do some minimal acting, secondary performers do the comic routines and humorous songs, the chorus sings, and no one dances except clearly designated dancers. These requirements make such shows attractive for productions presented by purely musical organizations, such as the school choir, because the acting and dancing demands are minimal and they show off what the musicians can do. However, practically all operettas demand a large, competent male chorus, which serves to discourage many of the same musical groups.

ANNIE
AGENT: Music Theatre
TYPE: book
PERIOD: 1930s
SET: drop
CAST: large
ATTRACTIONS: lots of parts for kids; extremely well-known material; wholesome family material
PROBLEMS: double casting generally necessary to save voice of young girl playing Annie; lots of sets; scenery and costumes more expensive than they look like at first glance; some significant differences from movie may affect expectations

ANYTHING GOES
AGENT: Tams-Witmark
TYPE: book (current version significantly rewritten from original)
PERIOD: 1930s
SET: drop
CAST: medium to large, flexible size chorus

ATTRACTIONS: collection of superb Cole Porter songs; revised book often very funny; orchestrated for jazz band rather than full orchestra
PROBLEMS: songs not as easy to sing as they sound; production numbers not very well integrated into book

BABES IN ARMS
AGENT: Rodgers & Hammerstein
TYPE: book
PERIOD: 1930s or "modern"
SET: drop
CAST: large
ATTRACTIONS: Rodgers and Hart music
PROBLEMS: silly "let's put on a show" book (now available in 1959 revision, improved but not all that much); lots of set and costume changes

THE BOY FRIEND
AGENT: Music Theatre
TYPE: book
PERIOD: 1920s
SET: three full-stage sets
CAST: medium
ATTRACTIONS: charming parody of twenties collegiate musicals; few demands on actors; pleasant music; little spectacle; minimal budget demands; songs spread among several principals
PROBLEMS: hard to balance performances to maintain the parody; audiences no longer aware of originals may miss most of jokes

BRIGADOON
AGENT: Tams-Witmark
TYPE: book
PERIOD: fantasy Scottish and modern
SET: drop
CAST: large (mostly chorus)
ATTRACTIONS: famous score; several nonsinging roles; dance can be confined to two people plus group folk dancing
PROBLEMS: kilts make the males very uncomfortable; opening scene and finale almost demand a scrim in addition to usual scenery pieces; female dancer must be ballerina, one principal a good, genuine tenor

BYE BYE BIRDIE
AGENT: Tams-Witmark
TYPE: book
PERIOD: late 1950s
SET: drop
CAST: large
ATTRACTIONS: lots of roles for teenagers; easy Elvis parody; songs generally easy to sing; costumes easy to make or find
PROBLEMS: lots of sets; much of dialogue dated and period jokes not always clear

CABARET
AGENT: Tams-Witmark
TYPE: book
PERIOD: early 1930s
SET: drop/unit mix
CAST: medium to large
ATTRACTIONS: several mature principals (very rare in musicals); vivid musical numbers; extremely theatrical production
PROBLEMS: scenery very complex; tone difficult to maintain; not at all like the movie (Sally in fact a smallish role) so expectations not always satisfied

CAMELOT
AGENT: Tams-Witmark
TYPE: book, with strong spectacle
PERIOD: medieval fairy tale
SET: drop
CAST: large
ATTRACTIONS: famous, attractive music; good acting roles; dance not too demanding
PROBLEMS: very expensive sets and costumes; predominantly male roles; only three developed characters, which makes it hard for many groups to justify the expense of full production

CARNIVAL!
AGENT: Tams-Witmark
TYPE: book
PERIOD: "modern" circus
SET: drop
CAST: large
ATTRACTIONS: excellent blend of naiveté and sophistication; circus setting provides lots of color as well as opportunity for specialty bits from performers; five or six really interesting roles
PROBLEMS: principals must act and sing convincingly; music for male and female leads very demanding; functioning magic tricks essential to plot; puppeteers and good puppets essential

CAROUSEL
AGENT: Rodgers & Hammerstein
TYPE: book
PERIOD: 1870s
SET: drop
CAST: large
ATTRACTIONS: every song a hit; moving book
PROBLEMS: some awkward set changes; dream scene demands ballerina; skilled male dancers required; principals must be good singer/actors

COMPANY
AGENT: Music Theatre
TYPE: book/ensemble
PERIOD: 1970s
SET: unit
CAST: small

ATTRACTIONS: terrific songs; adult wit and theme; well-balanced and interesting roles for all the cast

PROBLEMS: orchestral sound essential to success; plot not always obvious; difficult music for inexperienced singers; audiences tend to love or hate it with no middle ground; bed scene

DAMN YANKEES

AGENT: Music Theatre
TYPE: star
PERIOD: "modern" baseball
SET: drop
CAST: medium
ATTRACTIONS: easy costume and generally easy staging demands; story attractive to broad audience
PROBLEMS: almost all male cast; female "star" must be able to carry much of music and dance alone

DESERT SONG

AGENT: French
TYPE: operetta
PERIOD: Arab/Foreign Legion
SET: drop
CAST: large
ATTRACTIONS: lovely music; colorful costume and sets; one of most effective pieces of pure romance ever put on stage
PROBLEMS: singers must sing; strings essential in orchestra; book still has spells of unintentional silliness, especially at the end; romantic principals must actually look like romantic leads

THE FANTASTICKS

AGENT: Music Theatre
TYPE: ensemble with good book
PERIOD: "modern"
SET: bare stage with props
CAST: small
ATTRACTIONS: minimal sets and costume costs; famous good songs; no dance required
PROBLEMS: singers must sing well; only one female role; "rape" song often causes community problems despite the show's essential innocence

FIDDLER ON THE ROOF

AGENT: Music Theatre
TYPE: star with good book
PERIOD: Russian peasant, 1900
SET: drop
CAST: large
ATTRACTIONS: moving subject matter well realized
PROBLEMS: star role participates in almost every number; male dancers essential; original design and choreography essential to feel of the show (which means great demands on budget and dancers)

FUNNY GIRL
AGENT: Tams-Witmark
TYPE: star with some spectacle
PERIOD: 1920s and showgirl
SET: drop
CAST: large
ATTRACTIONS: spectacle; widely known material; generally good songs
PROBLEMS: Streisand vehicle forces Streisand expectations; staging sometimes clumsy; no way to trim budget on Ziegfeld scenes and retain look of show

A FUNNY THING HAPPENED ON THE WAY TO THE FORUM
AGENT: Music Theatre
TYPE: book with large star part
PERIOD: Ancient Rome
SET: single set
CAST: medium
ATTRACTIONS: very funny; easy to sing; no scenery changes; costumes comparatively inexpensive
PROBLEMS: few women's roles; much of its success depends on a principal actor audiences really like; a lot of sex jokes that may offend some audiences

GODSPELL
AGENT: Theatre Maximus
TYPE: ensemble/revue
PERIOD: clown, no period
SET: single set, almost bare stage
CAST: small
ATTRACTIONS: set and costumes can be done with almost no budget; all cast members get solos; subject matter (Christ's teaching and Last Supper) extremely broad interest; humor and imagination as well as sincerity
PROBLEMS: ensemble must be equally talented; religious aspects hard to balance in many communities (some see it as sacrilegious while others see it as too sectarian)

GREASE
AGENT: French
TYPE: ensemble
PERIOD: 1950s youth
SET: unit
CAST: medium to large, much flexibility possible
ATTRACTIONS: lots of roles for teenagers (none of them particularly demanding in skill); audiences in general love it even when (or perhaps especially when) it has a less than perfect production; costumes and sets can be done with low budget
PROBLEMS: bad productions happen easily because the parody elements are obvious and become repetitive without extremely inventive choreography; rock score demands a particularly good sound system

GUYS AND DOLLS
AGENT: Music Theatre
TYPE: book
PERIOD: 1950s adult

SET: drop
CAST: large
ATTRACTIONS: classic show with solid book and excellent characterizations; famous songs; minimal dance requirements
PROBLEMS: mostly male cast; scenery changes extensive; the peculiar slang very difficult for actors to speak well; top quality actor/singers needed for many roles; by contemporary standards a very long show

GYPSY
AGENT: Tams-Witmark
TYPE: star with considerable spectacle
PERIOD: 1920–1950
SET: drop
CAST: large
ATTRACTIONS: lots of roles; almost all singers and dancers are female; well-known show
PROBLEMS: sets and costumes complex and expensive; "striptease" background upsets some communities; star role demands a peculiar set of talents; enormous cast even by musical standards

HELLO, DOLLY!
AGENT: Tams-Witmark
TYPE: star with okay book
PERIOD: 1890s
SET: drop
CAST: medium
ATTRACTIONS: famous show; allows use of middle-aged star (fairly rare in musicals); dance can be quite simple or complex according to local needs
PROBLEMS: the show became a hit from one number and one performer and audiences don't quite know what to expect when that number is over; the book and music do not give the rest of the cast much support; strong chorus and dance demand on males

H.M.S. PINAFORE
AGENT: public domain
TYPE: operetta
PERIOD: 1880s
SET: single set
CAST: medium
ATTRACTIONS: good roles for quality singers; libretto still funny; Gilbert & Sullivan aficionados provide a solid base for cast and audience; no set or costume changes (costumes easily rentable); no dance; no royalties
PROBLEMS: singers must sing well and have good diction; Gilbert & Sullivan traditions raise demanding audience expectations about style of presentation; younger audiences and performers often find the music incomprehensible

THE KING AND I
AGENT: Rodgers & Hammerstein
TYPE: book with lots of spectacle
PERIOD: 1860s and Siamese

SET: drop
CAST: large
ATTRACTIONS: good and famous score; solid book; lots of roles for children
PROBLEMS: extremely expensive production; real actors needed in principal roles; dancers and choreographer must be skilled

KISMET
AGENT: Music Theatre
TYPE: operetta
PERIOD: Arabian Nights
SET: drop
CAST: large
ATTRACTIONS: gorgeous music; unusually good combination of romance, humor, and spectacle; probably the wittiest operetta book available
PROBLEMS: must have trained voices and a full orchestra; costumes and scenery not particularly complicated but very expensive

KISS ME, KATE
AGENT: Tams-Witmark
TYPE: book
PERIOD: "modern" and Italian Renaissance
SET: drop
CAST: medium to large depending on chorus used
ATTRACTIONS: Cole Porter songs; witty lyrics and dialogue; use of Shakespearean play-within-a-play suggests "culture" within a very entertaining frame
PROBLEMS: considering the premise, the staging is often slow and clumsy; most roles male (including all but one solo dancer); males often uncomfortable in Shakespearean costumes; principals must speak both casual American and Shakespearean dialogue

LI'L ABNER
AGENT: Tams-Witmark
TYPE: spectacle
PERIOD: cartoon strip hillbilly
SET: drop
CAST: large
ATTRACTIONS: lots of small, easy roles; costumes easy to make; dance and music relatively undemanding
PROBLEMS: hard to pull off book based on comic strip as simple rather than simpleminded; large number of crowd scenes demand much rehearsal; the cartoon look is the show (so as audiences forget the comic the show becomes less comprehensible)

LITTLE MARY SUNSHINE
AGENT: French
TYPE: operetta
PERIOD: "Canadian Northwest Mounties"
SET: drop
CAST: medium
ATTRACTIONS: witty parody of MacDonald-Eddy movies; low budget and technical requirements; no orchestra needed
PROBLEMS: trained singers essential; much of the parody elements no longer clear to audience or performers who cannot remember the old movie operettas

A LITTLE NIGHT MUSIC
AGENT: Music Theatre
TYPE: book
PERIOD: turn of the century
SET: drop
CAST: medium
ATTRACTIONS: no chorus or dancers; gorgeous music; extremely witty and intelligent book and lyrics
PROBLEMS: everyone must sing and act; strings in full orchestra essential; demands both theatrical and sexual sophistication from performers and audience; scenery relatively complex

MAN OF LA MANCHA
AGENT: Tams-Witmark
TYPE: book with star part
PERIOD: sixteenth century
SET: single set
CAST: medium
ATTRACTIONS: one set; limited dance; emotionally powerful and moving show
PROBLEMS: lots of men, few women; quality actor/singers required

THE MIKADO
AGENT: public domain
TYPE: operetta
PERIOD: traditional Japanese
SET: two full stage sets
CAST: medium
ATTRACTIONS: see *H.M.S. Pinafore*
PROBLEMS: Japanese costuming expensive and hard for performers to adjust to; for other problems see *H.M.S. Pinafore*

THE MUSIC MAN
AGENT: Music Theatre
TYPE: book with star part
PERIOD: 1910
SET: drop
CAST: large
ATTRACTIONS: quintessential Americana; lots of varied roles for all age groups; attractive music (including period barbershop songs)
PROBLEMS: real barbershop quartet essential; star male role demands an unusual song delivery; lots of crowd scenes to rehearse; more dance to stage than it looks like at first glance

MY FAIR LADY
AGENT: Tams-Witmark
TYPE: book
PERIOD: 1912 England
SET: drop
CAST: medium
ATTRACTIONS: famous classic show; wit, intelligence, sophistication; lovely songs; relatively limited dance

PROBLEMS: costumes and actors must be elegant; English accents and precise diction absolutely essential

OKLAHOMA!
AGENT: Rodgers & Hammerstein
TYPE: book
PERIOD: "cowboy"
SET: drop
CAST: large
ATTRACTIONS: classic songs; wholesome nostalgia; costumes easy to make; for dancers a real chance to shine
PROBLEMS: large number of classically trained dancers essential; show has a tendency to seem hokey if not treated absolutely sincerely; heavy acting/dancing demands on males

OLIVER!
AGENT: Tams-Witmark
TYPE: book
PERIOD: Dickensian England
SET: drop
CAST: large
ATTRACTIONS: solid book; lots of roles for children
PROBLEMS: many roles require children (who are hard to rehearse); few women's roles; extensive scenery and costume demands

ONCE UPON A MATTRESS
AGENT: Music Theatre
TYPE: book
PERIOD: fairytale medieval
SET: drop
CAST: medium
ATTRACTIONS: funny material; scenery and costume requirements relatively simple; dance eccentric but not terribly difficult
PROBLEMS: plot hinges on a number of illegitimate pregnancies that may offend some audiences; no hit songs to help publicity

PETER PAN
AGENT: French
TYPE: book
PERIOD: fairytale Edwardian
SET: drop
CAST: large
ATTRACTIONS: famous story; many roles for young performers; attractive to both child and adult audiences
PROBLEMS: fiendishly difficult staging including flying of several characters simultaneously and swordfights; special effects very demanding (Tinkerbell, house built on stage, etc.); animal costumes

THE PIRATES OF PENZANCE
AGENT: public domain
TYPE: operetta

PERIOD: 1880s
SET: two full stage sets
CAST: medium
ATTRACTIONS: see *H.M.S. Pinafore*
PROBLEMS: see *H.M.S. Pinafore. Note:* The recent New York revival completely rearranged the orchestral parts, modified or added songs, and for all practical purposes rewrote the characters and traditional business; if this is the show you wish to produce, scripts can be obtained from Music Theatre and royalty must be paid. By the same token, most groups face unusual audience expectations, as some will expect traditional Gilbert & Sullivan while others will expect this new version.

THE ROBBER BRIDEGROOM
AGENT: Music Theatre
TYPE: book/ensemble
PERIOD: 1790s Mississippi
SET: unit
CAST: medium
ATTRACTIONS: energy, wit, imagination in staging; simple scene and costume requirements; uses the chorus as a real acting ensemble to play many parts (including scenery at times), which has made it a favorite of colleges; blue-grass band for orchestra; lots of "movement" but not much "dance"
PROBLEMS: relatively unknown; "nude" scene and pregnancy upsets some audiences; physically demanding for all performers

SHOW BOAT
AGENT: Rodgers & Hammerstein
TYPE: book
PERIOD: 1880-1927
SET: drop
CAST: large
ATTRACTIONS: great music; classic mature book
PROBLEMS: enormous sets and many costumes over a long time period make it very expensive; real singers needed; for modern audiences a very long show with songs far between

THE SOUND OF MUSIC
AGENT: Rodgers & Hammerstein
TYPE: star
PERIOD: 1930s
SET: drop
CAST: medium to large as desired
ATTRACTIONS: wholesome show attractive to family audiences; parts for all ages of performers
PROBLEMS: a dozen sets; sometimes so sweet your teeth hurt; a star vehicle, but the star is not Julie Andrews, which leads to some odd audience expectation problems; although costumes seem simple, there are a lot of them

SOUTH PACIFIC
AGENT: Rodgers & Hammerstein
TYPE: book
PERIOD: World War II military and Polynesian

SET: drop
CAST: large
ATTRACTIONS: lots of roles; every song a hit; almost all dancers are female; serious, mature "message" along with romance and humor
PROBLEMS: lots of men required; staging gets really slow and awkward in Act II radio scenes; lots of sets; most contemporary casts will object to military haircuts; shower stall a harder effect than it looks

THE STUDENT PRINCE

AGENT: Tams-Witmark
TYPE: operetta
PERIOD: nineteenth-century German
SET: drop
CAST: medium to large, depending on chorus
ATTRACTIONS: pretty music
PROBLEMS: full orchestra and trained singers essential (especially difficult for male singers)

WEST SIDE STORY

AGENT: Music Theatre
TYPE: book
PERIOD: 1950s youth
SET: drop
CAST: large
ATTRACTIONS: youthful roles; vivid dramatic impact; great songs; no costume problems; interracial cast
PROBLEMS: real singer/dancer/actors needed; dance extremely important and demanding; probably the hardest orchestral score ever written for a musical

THE WIZARD OF OZ

AGENT: Tams-Witmark
TYPE: book
PERIOD: fairytale
SET: drop
CAST: large
ATTRACTIONS: lots of roles for kids; attractive to family audience; good songs; "just like the movie"
PROBLEMS: "just like the movie" does not always make for good or practical theatrical staging

YOU'RE A GOOD MAN, CHARLIE BROWN

AGENT: Tams-Witmark
TYPE: ensemble revue
PERIOD: cartoon modern
SET: unit
CAST: small
ATTRACTIONS: very simple set and costumes; low-budget; no dance; piano only score; characters and many scenes immediately familiar
PROBLEMS: works best in very small theatre, otherwise practically indestructible

Index